To
Jay Efrei;
with my best wishes,
Alexander Kra[?]wick

HUMANIZING
the
PSYCHIATRIC
HOSPITAL

Alexander Gralnick, M.D.

EDITOR

*Associate Clinical Professor of Psychiatry,
New York Medical College and
Medical Director of High Point Hospital,
Port Chester, New York*

in collaboration with

Frank G. D'Elia, M.D.

Maurice H. Greenhill, M.D.

Guillermo del Castillo, M.D.

Rustu Yemez, M.D.

Faruk Turker, M.D.

Peter Schween, M.D.

Walmor L. Berger, M.D.

Leatrice Styrt Schacht, M.A.

Murray Blacker, Ph.D.

Edwin L. Rabiner, M.D.

Morton F. Reiser, M.D.

Harriet L. Barr, Ph.D.

Daniel Zawel, M.S.

HUMANIZING the PSYCHIATRIC HOSPITAL

Jason Aronson   New York

Gralnick, Alexander
   Humanizing the Psychiatric Hospital
© 1975 Jason Aronson Inc. New York

ISBN: 0-87668-158-5

Library of Congress Catalog Number: 74-6961

All royalties from this book will be donated to "The Gralnick Foundation"

Dedicated to

Stephen P. Jewett, M.D. (1883–1971)

Mentor, teacher, colleague, good friend

and

Faruk Turker, M.D. (1921–1971)

Student, loyal and devoted member of

our Staff

Both very Human beings.

Contents

III. CLINICAL RESEARCH

Preface

"Humanizing the Psychiatric Hospital." At first this title may perplex the reader. Does a hospital where the emotionally troubled person goes to reacquire mental health need to be humanized? Must we not take for granted that a human aspect exists and is experienced by the patient, every day, every hour, constantly and without reservation?

These are legitimate and healthy questions. But the answer is that this humanizing endeavor has to be stressed, increased, and not at all taken for granted. Although it is to be assumed that all administrations of psychiatric hospitals wanted to offer to the patient a humane milieu, three factors slowed the process of humanization. The first is the nature of mental illness, that at times transforms the human being into an individual who is occasionally antisocial and frequently inconsiderate of social expectations. The second is tradition. The hospital used to be a place where undesirable people, potentially dangerous or of public scandal, were relegated. The third factor refers to the methods of treatment, like forced custodial care, restraint, or even psychosurgery and electric shock treatment, which did not shine for their humane qualities, even if they were the only effective methods at the time they were used.

Fortunately these three factors are things of the past. Vestiges of them continue to linger, but their impact is constantly decreased by virtue of all the humanizing efforts. The mental patient is no longer seen as a less human member of the human community but as a person who has suffered more, at times because of society, and who must be encouraged to trust society again. The hospital is not an asylum or a sanctuary for the unwanted, but a regenerative center for people who are wanted back as soon as possible. Although the old methods of treatment are still used in rare cases, the majority of patients are nowadays treated by a combination of drug therapy and psychotherapy. The latter helps the patient to lose his conflicts, to acquire a new self-image, new hopes, and new ways with which to face life in a more rewarding manner.

This book will clearly show how such humanizing effect is put into practice at High Point Hospital. Whether the aim is to formulate a clinical theory or a clinical application, or a research, the reader will recognize that a scientific aim of daring quality is always accompanied by a human side which in the majority of instances touches deeply and quickly heals.

SILVANO ARIETI, M.D.

Clinical Professor of Psychiatry
New York Medical College

Foreword

This book is the succeeding volume to a work which demonstrated that the organizational structure and administrative functions of a psychiatric hospital had a therapeutic influence upon the process of illness and its outcome. The focus upon the therapeutic effect of the hospital itself in a clinical organization which was that aware of its own influences naturally led to a realization of its own anti-therapeutic potentials.

For several years High Point Hospital has been involved in evaluation studies of its practices and theoretical approach. These have been published in a number of theoretical and position papers by the medical director and his coworkers and a smaller number of significant articles presenting data and research design. This book represents the second collation of such publications and is organized to present its efforts in grappling with such anti-therapeutic forces as dehumanizing effects within a hospital environment, whether it be this or any other hospital.

What in reality is being considered are those subliminal influences within the hospital social structure and its therapeutic programs which are negatively interpersonal and may lead to unnecessary suffering, obstruction to improvement and recovery, and injustice. These are called "dehumanizing" effects by the editor, implying that they reduce the individual, subject him to insensibilities, and traumatize him within a protective and nurturing environment. His message is that ongoing identification and evaluation of dehumanizing effects makes possible not only their management but also leads to the designing of humanizing methods as therapeutic techniques. This requires not only periodic scanning of administrative policies and therapeutic relationships among and between staff and patients at conferences and at meetings of the Board of Governors, but also a built-in ever-present perceptiveness of the high priority of humaneness and human values.

Such a work is timely in this day of technocracy when only a few voices are heard speaking out against the impersonal and dehumanizing atmosphere of computerized medical science. It is also well-timed and significant in a period when under the guise that psychiatric hospitals are for the most part obsolescent and inhuman, it is claimed that their eradication is necessary and is indeed underway. Is this fact or is this one more of the many psychiatric fashions which have come and gone? What we read here in this volume makes us consider that the decline of the psychiatric hospital in favor of current plans or lack of plans for community management may be just another form of dehumanization of the patient.

MAURICE H. GREENHILL, M.D.

Professor of Psychiatry
Albert Einstein College of Medicine

Introduction

The concept this book advances is an inevitable outgrowth of the practice of milieu therapy and the structuring of the inhospital psychotherapeutic community. New theory evolves from gathering experience and the changing techniques it dictates. New perspectives are also a natural accompaniment of this phenomenon. The "hospital community" idea and the concept of the psychiatric hospital as a therapeutic instrument has increasingly led to the perception of the importance of the human relationships existing therein. Their nature came to seem as important as a particular medical modality itself. Consequently the study of these relationships between patients and between patients and staff was deemed essential. It also became imperative to structure these human relationships, to mold their character so that, as parameters of an environment, they would have a health-producing effect. The critical importance of values came to the fore. In simple terms, the way people treated each other—how "human" they were—took on a significance of increasing proportions and opened new horizons.

The challenge, however, was to give the practice of hospital psychiatry a social perspective without sacrificing its clinical nature. The disease entity with which we dealt was medical, but, as with other such entities, the aid of other disciplines was essential. Therefore the social factors which affected it became important to its understanding and resolution. In other words, it is as important to know the social aspects of mental disorders, their cure and prevention, as it is to know and control the social aspects of drug addiction or venereal disease. Since a psychiatric hospital is a social structure, one must be mindful of all these considerations if he is to understand and resolve the direction the mental disorder takes within the confines of that society.

This requires an awareness of the human qualities of the diseased individual, an acceptance of the importance of improving those qualities, and a method—or social system—to promote the patient's humanization.

It has been about five years since thoughts about the humanizing potential of the psychiatric hospital began to percolate in our minds. At times the notion was nebulous, and doubts about its validity assailed us. This will be obvious from a reading of our first effort to commit these thoughts to writing in the paper, "The Humanizing Influence of the Psychiatric Hospital," which appears as Chapter 3 in this book. As a consequence, there was no specially concentrated emphasis on the theme or a conscious continuity given to it in our writings. On closer inspection, however, and in preparation for this book, we recognized that elements of the larger theme, both in theory and in application, had been and were recurring in our papers. Our hope, then, is that the reader will pick these up, especially with the assistance of the heretofore unpublished chapter, "Humanization and the Inpatient Therapeutic Process," which attempts to highlight these features. We found that we had gone so far as to examine the pros and cons of the value of our very existence in the paper, "The Proprietary Hospital: To Be or Not to Be."

The discussion first appeared to lend itself to chronological treatment, but it soon appeared that the subject would fall quite naturally into three categories: clinical theory, clinical studies, and clinical research. Chapter 6 will aid in giving some historical perspective to the total effort.

At any one point a hospital is a cross-section of the efforts of all those who have participated in its technical and theoretical development. This has always been true of High Point Hospital and is particularly true now as it ventures into new areas.

This book is a second series of papers containing the expressions of those who have had a particular human experience in a single, changing hospital system. It holds and describes the germ of a theme born almost a generation ago and developed through the succeeding years of a unique clinical experience with the mentally ill. This book expresses a conceptualization for the understanding and treatment of psychopathology, particularly the most common form, schizophrenia. As developed to this point, the concept is the culmination of the thinking of the many who engaged in and contributed to the development of a special system now represented by High Point Hospital. Their esprit de corps and ability to continuously reach a consensus on arising issues were the keys to our accomplishment.

I would like to express my thanks to all the authors and to the journal editors who permitted republication of the papers. As medical director of the hospital from which these papers emanate, I give thanks to all in the supporting professional and nonprofessional services whose dedication has made our medical achievements possible. Much appreciation is also expressed for the constant support of our Board of Governors: Maurice Greenhill, M.D., chairman; Silvano Arieti, M.D.; Bernard D. Fischman, esq.; and L. Clovis Hirning, M.D. No end of thanks is also due and given to my faithful and loyal personal secretary, Fanny Jane Holmes who worked so diligently in the preparation of the manuscript and related details.

cally they have been rejected by the clinician. The hospital psychiatrist, particularly, tends to think in terms of promptly freeing the patient of his symptoms and returning him to society. This has become especially true as the belief (or *myth,* since it has by no means been proven) has grown to the point of being taken as fact that the patient is better off "in the community." Therefore, it becomes quite a task to initiate thinking in terms of the longer-range goal of "humanizing" the patient and to formulate acceptable reasons to justify this area as one of legitimate concern for psychiatrists. The implication is that patients are "dehumanized," at least to some extent, which adds fuel to the fire that already scars the patient with stigma if he is "merely" mentally ill. Yet we hear on all sides not only that mental hospitals are dehumanizing, but that society is sick and is dehumanizing its citizens. It does not take a great step, therefore, to wonder whether our patients, in addition, suffered a dehumanizing process before their hospitalization. Further, if the dehumanizing experiences affect their illness, there would seem to be some logic in exposing them to humanizing ones in a hospital setting.

On reflection, then, there might really be an urgent need to study the relation between dehumanizing experiences and the formation of mental illness, as well as the effect of humanizing experiences in arresting and reversing the psychotic process. This logic seems consistent with the relatively simple concept that if mental illness is born in a traumatic, or "sick," social setting, then we should be able to overcome it in a "healthy" setting. A mental institution, strange as it may seem, can be a healthy environment! It is there where patients get well, while it is "on the outside" (where they had all their freedoms and liberties) that they became ill. We are inevitably faced, then, with considering the humanizing elements of a psychiatric hospital. What are they? What else should they be? How are they introduced into and maintained in the hospital? How do they *humanize* the patient? How does this result effect an alleviation of symptoms and fortify the patient against the dehumanizing influences he will once more face when released into "society"? It is much easier to formulate the questions than their answers.

Chapter 1
Humanization and the
Inpatient Therapeutic Process

In this book we have delineated the growth and evolution of our concepts and therapeutic efforts at High Point Hospital. As a series of studies it demonstrates a theme consistent with factors which have a humanizing effect on people. It considers the "humanization" of a patient as the concern of the hospital psychiatrist, that his domain extends beyond the mere "treatment" of the patient's symptoms. Though he is a person, the patient's "human" attributes may no longer be taken for granted as being present in sufficient quantity and quality, or in other ways solely the field for study by other professionals. The writer, a psychiatrist, resolves that he will not stray into areas of a philosophical nature and out of the clinical context, particulary as he is always surrounded by criticism highlighting the rarely defined "dehumanizing" effect of hospitalization. Of necessity, then, he enters the field to clarify the questions thereby raised, both for himself and for others. Nevertheless, it seems well nigh impossible to evade the philosophical and moral overtones implicit in the subject matter, because the field of psychiatry has been increasingly invaded by others. Among these are the philosopher, sociologist, religious leader, and most particularly, the civil libertarian lawyer zealously protecting the patient's constitutional liberties and "human" rights against society's unaware agent, the psychiatrist. Beyond all this is the fact that the psychiatrist is a flesh-and-blood being who is inseparable from his own human value systems which operate in all of his considerations regarding treatment. His own degree of humanization is not an absolute.

Philosophical and moral questions are "strange"; histori-

3

PART ONE
CLINICAL THEORY

It is a fact that many hospitals, if not a majority, are hardly what we would like them to be. This should come as no surprise to anyone, for psychiatric hospitals are products of and reflections of the society in which they exist, and that society is hardly what we would like it to be. Probably one problem will not likely be solved without solving the other, yet some patients do improve in all hospitals. I would therefore surmise that even in the worst hospital, therapeutic relationships are at work, and perhaps even humanizing ones. It is just that we have neither looked for nor sought to define and develop them to a high degree. This may now be the psychiatric task facing us and the one to which we must eventually address ourselves. This chapter—and this book—is an effort in that direction.

In their book, *The Humanization Processes,*[1] the authors make statements and present concepts which are germane to the thesis of this book. For instance, Hamblin, the senior author, says: "Many assume that an infant, at birth, is human in the full sense of the word. He is potentially human, but those most human qualities have to be acquired or developed over a score of years in a human society with an extant culture. Our definition of *human* includes that which is humane or truly civilized, and we focus on the humane processes of humanization. It is our feeling that children can learn to be humane only in a social environment which is itself humane."

Though the authors of *The Humanization Processes* are all sociologists, they describe their work as "neither pure sociology nor pure psychology, but a blend of both." While they admit to following the "learning psychologist," they indicate their differences in that they "tend to think in exchange theoretical terms—and are always talking about structuring and restructuring social exchanges," thus indicating that human behavior changes only if present types of social exchange systems are modified. Using the language of the sociologist, they seem to be saying what we have been doing in our hospital and stating in our papers. On the basis of continuing clinical experience through the years, we have structured and restructured, modified and remodeled the manner in which patients as individuals and groups are related to each other and to the professional staff (social exchange systems). With this technique we believe we have not merely alleviated symptoms but altered personalities and contributed to the humanization process.

Hamblin says that their experiments "demonstrate the intimate relationship between the structure of social exchange systems and acculturation." They show that in order to change man's behavior it is usually necessary to change the structure of the social exchange systems under which man operates. After postulating the theory they call the "inadvertent exchange theory of deviancy," Hamblin states further: "Our experimental results show that tragedy may be avoided if the child is placed in an alternative social structure where he is rewarded systematically and meaningfully for behaving normally, and where he earns nothing for behaving deviantly." We would like to think that this use of an "alternative social structure" also coincides with our idea of the hospital as a useful alternative system structured to overcome the pathology produced in the larger society and that this, too, is manifest in the present book. In some respects, High Point Hospital has also been "experimental," in that it has continuously studied and altered its social system to meet the changing nature and demands of its inhabitants.

On a global scale, Hamblin believes that our poorly devised social exchange systems have failed to condition man to live productively and happily. On the contrary, they may have conditioned him to live the way he generally does: exploitatively, aggressively, and destructively. On the scientific level, then, Hamblin sees the scientist as having to learn (1) how structured social systems condition those who live in them, and (2) how to structure social systems so that they will benefit everyone concerned. The latter aim has been our particular concern in hospital psychiatry, the goal we have been trying to reach with our work.

I would like particularly to emphasize Hamblin's declaration that as scientists, his group empathizes with those they are studying and allows their feelings to show, "because to hide them would be dishonest and unwise." He says, further, that while one is trained to be "cold and dispassionate" as a scientist, "one is not required to be cold and dispassionate about mankind. Scientists, as well as other people, are at their worst when they are unfeeling for others." I take this quotation to strongly suggest the use of one's emotions and value systems in the study and treatment of patients and therefore to be in accord with what we have been trying to convey in both our previous and our present book.

In discussing their "structured exchange theory," Hamblin and his coworkers have better expressed the essence of our own labors. They say that their work documents "the theory that social learning environments are structured as exchanges—and that the fundamental social exchange is always between two parties—one taking an initiator role and the other a reciprocator role." This is exactly what we believe has transpired in the exchanges between our professional and patient groups.

The changes we have seen in the symptoms, nature, and human qualities of our patients in the structured, clinical social system we have devised is again better stated by Hamblin et al. as sociologists. They say:

> Social exchanges are structured if they are worked repetitively and if reciprocation is patterned enough to be reliably characterized by a rule by sensitive observers. Structured exchanges are important because they, not transient exchanges, produce social learning and social conditioning. Social exchanges become structured in several ways—the vast majority are structured implicitly, as it were, without verbal negotiations. People are generally unaware of the thousands of implicitly structured exchanges in which they are involved every day—they are often oblivious of the learning and conditioning that occurs as a result.

As is documented by the articles in this book, the social system of High Point Hospital is so structured that exchanges are "characterized by rule"; they undoubtedly produce the "social learning and conditioning" which we, as psychiatrists, have otherwise described in our own language as the process of overcoming resistance and symptoms, getting well, maturing, the process of rehabilitation and reconstruction, and the process of personality change. Now we are inclined to say that the proper "structured exchanges" promote some "humanization" in the patient. Incidentally, the thinking of Hamblin and Lennard[2] seems quite similar, the first speaking of "social exchange systems" needing change and the second of "social relatedness" which needs revision if man is to learn to live with himself more humanely.

Acculturation refers to the "accumulative learning effects" which involve the "acquisition of the behavior and thought patterns of a particular culture." It includes the transformation of "the infant into a functional adult with the ability to relate to other adults, to solve problems, and to exercise a measure of control over self and others. It is only when the normal acculturation processes go awry that the disorders appear . . .," but "in their normal form, the acculturation processes are, in fact, synonymous with the humanization processes." These quotes, which are also from Hamblin, express our thinking and attempts, if not achievement, to have the patient acculturate to the hospital social system and thereby be transformed into a "functional adult." We believe we are at least occasionally successful to the point that the process takes on a certain normality which leads to a patient's "humanization." It appears to us that the ultimate goal of the hospital of the future, or any treatment system substituted for it, should be to achieve regular success of this kind.

It is shocking to a psychiatrist to face the fact that, other than his speculation, he knows little, if anything, scientifically about what makes one mentally healthy. It is sad enough to accept how uncertain we are of the real causes of mental illness, let alone how inadequate we are at coping on a significant scale with the proliferating problems the mentally sick present us. Imagine the task we assume, then, in undertaking the humanizing of the person with a disordered mind and the effect such an undertaking may have on us; yet we can no longer shrink from the subject, difficult as the task may appear.

Some students of man save themselves the dilemma by easy surrender to or total involvement in the cytoarchitecture of man's brain. Pribram simply states: "What makes man human is his brain. This brain is obviously different from those of non-human primates.'' When he asks himself whether these characteristics of the brain ''determine the humanness of man,'' however, he comments: ''This paper cannot give an answer to this question, for the answer is not known.'' Yet seek it we must! Man is now reaching the moon and even Venus in his quest for their secrets and through them, knowledge of the origins of the planet he inhabits. He cannot evade the lesser task of discovering what humanizes him, for only that knowledge will permit him to save from utter destruction the very world and its inhabitants whose origins he wishes to understand.

In early September 1972 some 3,000 theologians met at an international congress on ''Religion and the Humanizing of Man.'' The chairman of the congress, Dr. James M. Robinson,[3] a professor of religion, stated: ''We pushed toward a new focus—the humanizing of man.'' One would have thought that this had always been the objective of religion, but apparently not. He stated further: ''At a time when the place of religion is far from clear, the urgent need to humanize mankind is thoroughly apparent. . . . The Congress presupposes that religion is meant to grapple . . . with this life.''

One may guess that this burgeoning interest in the humanization of man and its processes grows from the frightening conditions of prolonged war, the polarization of peoples, the rampant violence and terror, starvation, obvious environmental destruction, the hydrogen bomb's potential to destroy everybody, and the apparent neverending conflicts somewhere in the world. It is as though men were beginning to sense their plight and thus gain insight into a madness which brings them to the brink of destruction. With it, there would seem to be an awareness by man that he must look to himself for salvation—to some capacity still there, still capable of birth in him even in this ''sick society.'' The ability can only be that of discovering the origins of and actual achievement of ''humanization.'' The process is not unlike that which is occurring in the field of psychiatry as psychiatrists sense themselves being overwhelmed by the magnitude of their problems. The subject of ''dehumanization'' and ''humanization'' comes increasingly to the fore. We must also sense the importance of decent values and humanization to the prophylaxis and therapy of mental illness in all its manifestations.

In our speculations as psychiatrists and in our studies designed to "prove" which conditions promote emotional stability, if not mental health, we point to essential home and family conditions; they are purported by us as critically important to the formation of a "decent" or "humane" individual. More often we base our conclusions on the apparent absence of these conditions from the lives of those we study and treat, namely, the mentally ill. It is a well-known fact that we give little time to the study of the mentally healthy and the origins of this fortunate state. When we do, and include a consideration of what makes one more humanized than another, we frequently point to a number of factors. Upon close study of the articles in this book, which at first glance may seem disparate, these factors are shown to be a constant theme of the psychiatric hospital.

If an analogy may be drawn with the parent-child relationship—or, for that matter, with any relationship in which one affects another—there are several features we select which may have a positive (healthy or humanizing) effect. In the case of the infant we say that the process with the parents is one of acculturation, but in later relations we do not characterize them this way, although it would be appropriate to do so with patients who suddenly and for prolonged periods find themselves plunged into new relationships in what is a rather different social structure. In our experience this is especially true of the schizophrenic patient.

These qualities may be enumerated without our knowing the order of their importance in the humanizing process. To begin with, such relationships need stability, structure, and constancy, accompanied by flexibility and dependability. They require a large element of conscious study of one by the other to acquire understanding of and sensitivity to one another's respective needs. Only by acquiring such awareness can the needs of each be satisfied and gratification felt by the giver. Naturally, positive motivation must be present from the start, although this is probably learned in the process of living under conditions which evoke such attitudes. For the moment the exact nature of these conditions is unknown, or if it is, certainly not widely enough accepted to bring them into universal effectiveness.

The factors mentioned above are evident in the articles that follow. Those of care and concern for the patient and devotion to the positive treatment of him as a human being, and not merely as a "patient," are equally clear. There is plentiful evidence of strong emotional investment in the patient's life, his program, and the goal of successful treatment. There is self-criticism and constant self-evaluation on the part of the professional team—certainly no complacency. There is a constant search for a better way of living within the social system of the hospital, as well as a willingness to restructure in order to secure that result.

While the welfare and human development of the patient are the personnel's main aim, these are not seen as being accomplished by showering him with "love" and "freedom" to do as he wishes. Instead, we believe that the path to achieving the patient's health and "humanization" lies in the exercise of a firm though flexible approach based on our acknowledged better awareness of what he and his illness require. This is accompanied by patience and persistence in the face of the patient's resistance and in an atmosphere of protecting the patient's best interests, even though our ideas about them may differ from those of the patient and his family.

These features lend a sureness and stability to the hospital environment which are, in turn, important to the patient's progress and acculturation. Through experience, High Point Hospital has developed its mores, principles, and current system of values. It has become a society whose "exchange systems" are governed by rules. In other words, it has acquired its own laws. At the same time, we are aware that our hospital is only a reflection of the larger society which determines the degree of humanization—or the lack of it—in its inhabitants. We believe, however, that a hospital should contain those more desirable features of society which tend to humanize the individual. We hope that the articles which follow will uphold our belief that High Point Hospital has an abundance of identifiable elements which foster the patient's humanization.

REFERENCES

1. Hamblin, R. L., D. Buckholdt, D. Ferritor, M. Kozloff, and L. Blackwell. *The humanization processes: a social, behavioral analysis of children's problems*. New York: Wiley, 1971.

2. Lennard, H. L., and A. Bernstein. *Patterns in human interaction*. San Francisco: Jossey-Bass, 1969.

3. Robinson, J. M. Religion and the humanizing of man. *New York Times*, Sept. 9, 1972, p. 30.

Chapter 2
Social Forces and Patient Progress in the Psychotherapeutic Community

in collaboration with Frank G. D'Elia, M.D.

In a real sense social conditions are the determinants of psychiatric illness. Aberrations are bred under conditions of impoverishment of the quality and quantity of human relationships. This is to say, where there exists major psychopathology, there has existed some early deprivation of human emotional interaction vitally essential to the healthy growth and development of the personality. We may speculate that such impoverishment occurred early in the life of the victim as the result of certain human traits in those to whom his psychic development was first entrusted, namely, malevolence, misguided goodwill, or sheer inadvertence.

The conditions under which reparation is possible must accordingly be social. To control the progress of pathology, if not to reverse it entirely, we must first establish social conditions which will be either remedial in themselves or facilitate the operation of other therapies. Unable to reconstruct the society wherein illness was bred, we turn to the establishment of small psychiatric hospital societies. These remedial societies must ultimately be as enriched as the social anlage of the psychotic was impoverished. They must be as devoid as we can humanly make them of malevolence, uninformed benevolence, and negligence and as enriched as we can make them in all the healthy resources of human temperament.

13

Some would say that optimal conditions in such a model psychiatric society are therapeutic in themselves; others would say that these are merely the conditions under which other forms of therapy may best be done.[1-6] It is a moot point, but we believe that it remains for us to discover whether among these hospital conditions there are common "human" denominators which, in fact, account for the successes we see in approaches that differ from each other in other technical respects.

In considering what a psychiatric hospital community must be in order to be therapeutic, perhaps it might be more easily conceptualized in terms of what it must not be. It must not be, for example, a sterile and unproductive "back ward" aggregation of unrelated beings overseen by a lonely and distant attendant. This is not a "human" society. It lacks the attributes of mutuality which characterize normal human behavior.

We agree with Opler[7] that the human personality is the combined product of certain inherent potentials greatly modified by its social experiences. Personality aberrations are likewise a product of the vicissitudes of human interplay and interaction. The things that people do with and to each other affect them in beneficial and adverse ways. Human interaction, therefore, contains both the secrets of the etiology of psychopathology and the key to psychotherapy. We believe that emotional felicity in man is attained not by feeling *alone* and *against,* but by feeling *part of* and *allied with.* We believe that man may be a social animal, and that asocial, antisocial, and dyssocial states are not necessarily inevitable or irremediable. The health of a society can be gauged by the prevalence of certain forces and human values which tend to integrate and coordinate it against the pressures which tend to divide and disorganize it into the encapsulated and the estranged.

The psychiatrist is called to man's assistance when he strays from usual reaction norms. Our profession has utilized drugs and physiological procedures for the most part, though latter-day psychiatry has turned to the psychological and now social aspects of treatment. In doing so we have continued to house our sicker patients in institutions, but with increasing recognition of the need to draw upon disciplines other than the strictly medical.

Some psychiatric hospitals are no longer places where only physical methods of treatment are administered. Neither are they comfortable environments where solely humanitarian concepts are applied instead of, or in addition to, physiological procedures. Nor are they some mechanical combination of these approaches. They are, instead, social structures with their own mores and methods of living which are highly coordinated and integrated so that they may, of and by themselves, serve a therapeutic role.

There is reason to believe that by their very nature the social relationships existing in a psychiatric hospital affect the patient either in a negative or positive fashion. Social factors may be therapeutic or antitherapeutic. It is incumbent upon us, therefore, to determine and identify them so that the therapeutic may be reduplicated anywhere and the antitherapeutic eliminated. This has been the aim of our own hospital. It has permitted us to continue to introduce and maintain social factors thought to be of a therapeutic nature. Originally this was done in an almost unconscious fashion. Otherwise, factors have been introduced deliberately and their therapeutic effect tested by trial and error. By now we believe we have a number which we can identify and describe.

A similar process has been going on in psychoanalytic office practice. Therapists of differing persuasions and methods achieve good results. Each seeks and claims that "insight" helps his patient. The insight, however, that one therapist gives differs from the insight of another. The awareness is of a totally different nature. Yet the patients of both get well. This phenomenon can best be understood by defining the factors common to each treatment situation, namely, what is going on in the social environment of the persons involved. Factors of this nature are now being identified as the determinants which are therapeutic in their effect.

It seems today that too often almost any new way of treating a patient which is nonphysiologic is soon called an earmark of the therapeutic community. The "open-door policy," "day hospital," and "night hospital" are examples. Anything which makes life easier and more comfortable for the patient is introduced as a mark of the therapeutic community, as is anything which gives him more "freedom" and saves him the so-called indignities of the "traditional" hospital. Any environment which gives the patient little cause for complaint is "the therapeutic community." Any hospital which is "like home," or the way home should have been in the eyes of the psychiatrist, is the therapeutic community. An environment which is peaceful and permits leisure time, pleasures, and freedom from pressure is "the therapeutic community." Particularly, anything akin to the kindly and humane approach is considered therapeutic. Naturally, much depends on what one believes is *humane* and really decent treatment of the human being.

Anything which gives the patient status and an equal role is described as an element of the therapeutic community, particularly if it permits him to engage in conducting the affairs of the hospital. Daily ward meetings, therefore, between patients, nurses, and doctors are deemed ingredients of the therapeutic community.[8]

In many of these situations, however, the patient is given a role in which he may assume that he is other than an ill person, with the result that what was therapeutic in intention is antitherapeutic in effect. Thus might the patient be aided by the approach of those in authority in his efforts to evade facing the reality of his true status, namely, that he is an ill person. And yet the therapeutic community must be geared to dispel any breath of ignominy which may attach to the role of patient without obscuring the reality of this role. His feeling of significance in the therapeutic community should derive mainly from his living the role of patient, and neither doctor nor patient should lose sight of this. The therapeutic effect which follows the feeling of significant status should come from such treatment of him as conveys that he, as a patient, is the sole object of our concern and that all personnel are devoted to his welfare. The mechanics of ward meetings are less important. The hospital staff must realize, further, that their satisfaction and significance as members of the hospital community derive only from the presence of the patient and the theme that *his* welfare is of central significance to the community. In this context, then, ward meetings are no more vital than a host of other activities which may also convey this therapeutic theme.

Broadening the position of the therapist to that of a social role enhances his effectiveness in a therapeutic community. We recognize the therapist as a "social reinforcement agent,"[9] and we strive structurally to use his inherent skill in the greater social community—that is, our hospital community[10]—as contrasted to his individual psychotherapy with the patient. To the extent that we do this, to that extent are we fostering the therapeutic community hospital. In this context, then, we must be aware that diverting the hospital psychiatrist into the extramural community dilutes his role in the intramural community and thereby minimizes his opportunity to promote the therapeutic community aspects of his hospital. The point is, if we place our doctors out in the community too much, they lose much opportunity to play their proper role within the hospital and to devote ample time to the patient and the social community of the hospital. How must patients feel if, much of the time, the doctors responsible for their care are elsewhere? If it is really important for the patient to feel that he is the hub of the hospital, and this is therapeutic, he is going to feel incidental otherwise. This suggests an obvious disadvantage to the patient in an institution devoted mainly to training and research where he may feel secondary to a larger purpose.

By the same token, however, the psychiatrist who has really learned the principles of the therapeutic community in hospital practice is a more able exponent and practitioner of these principles when he does enter the extramural community practice of psychiatry. In other words, there is much the true hospital therapeutic community can demonstrate to, and for, the use of society. It need not be some anachronism—some artificial, undesirable life setting to which the patient is removed because society cannot take care of him for the moment. Hospitals should be communities which encourage society to take a positive and affirmative attitude when faced with hospitalizing one of its members. Hospitalization should not be by default, but by appropriate choice.

The present trend toward "community psychiatry" is perhaps an index and reflection of the degree to which mental hospitals have failed in their task and society itself has failed to assist in the complete development of their therapeutic potential. To the extent that hospitals become therapeutic communities, to that extent will the stress on community psychiatry be diminished. The hospital, and not the community, is really the place where appropriate patients should be treated, and for sufficiently long periods of time. Our task is to make hospitals what they should be. The community is where the illness was generated and perpetuated and therefore not necessarily the place in which the patient should be treated in his acute illness—unless, of course, we are prepared to change his community. It would be easier, to be sure, to change and improve the hospital.

When ill, the patient should be moved to a healthier section of society. The hospital should be that portion which is a distillate of the best, psychiatrically speaking, that society has to offer. This is perhaps what society has always dimly been asking. Unfortunately, it has not made the hospitals to fit the bill. On the contrary, many have been worse sections of society. Our aim should now be to form them into psychotherapeutic communities. The mentally ill are patients—and patients at appropriate times belong in proper hospitals. This is the logic to which we must subscribe.

We may ask ourselves whether the present state of community programs, short-term treatment regimes, and psychiatric units in general hospitals are really the "hospitals" of the future or our tacit admission that we cannot better fit the real hospital to the task. Are we loathe to face and admit wherein we really have failed, evading the real issue, namely, the perfection of the psychiatric hospital itself? Are we in psychiatry again grasping at the new, as a drowning man grasps at straws, before we have freely and fully tested the old? Are the present innovations being welcomed as the panacea, replacing the older ideas still untried, only to be succeeded in turn by the next "ultimate answer"? Are we so knowledgeable and successful in our field? Are we so learned that we can now afford to think in terms of discarding our hospitals? Would this be a sign of our advancement or an indication of our abject ignorance?

Among the factors affecting patient progress positively in a hospital is good communication. It must be maintained not only between the patient and doctor, but between the patients as a group and the doctors as a group. Communication, however, is synonymous with understanding. Since understanding between the sick and the well, let alone the well and the well, is not easily or instantly achieved, the therapeutic community must allow for a continuing process of communication and exchange which achieves the goal of mutual trust and respect for the role of each one as an individual and responsible member of his group.

The psychotic patient, as a rule, is so distrustful that the hospital's social structure must permit a process which constantly combats his distrust. Any factor which promotes such an achievement, and is built into the social structure, then is "therapeutic." The techniques, of course, may vary from individual psychotherapy to group discussions to patient bull sessions to frequent patient-medical staff contacts and exchanges of opinions. The more such levels of communication, the better. The more freely patients are in contact with each other and with skilled personnel, particularly in activities designed to evoke, explore, and overcome those emotional problems which promote distrust and isolation, the better for the patient. The more opportunity the patient has to know the minutiae of his sick personality, the better his chance to alter his ways of relating in a healthy direction. The more highly developed the understanding of the psychiatrist and the many professionals and nonprofessionals who assist him about the quality and nature of what is essential to communicate, the more likely is this communication system to serve its purpose successfully. The significance to the ultimate therapeutic goal of what is communicated is as important as the quality of the communication system itself.

As a supplement to common understanding there must be a mutuality of goals. Here again, the contrasting aims the patient has for himself must be brought into harmony with those of the psychiatrist. Fortunately for the patient, there is a difference between his original goals and our ultimate goals for him. However, the therapeutic community must help him realize this in the areas of everyday hospital experience additional to his psychotherapeutic sessions. This is the essence of the "total" 24-hour-a-day treatment model. To the extent that the hospital maintains the necessary mechanics to permit this, to that extent does it possess an essential therapeutic social factor. However, as the hospital's social structure becomes more complex, and those who come into meaningful relation with the patient become more numerous, it becomes perhaps quite as critically important that these others, though nonprofessional, also possess an increasing degree of understanding and agreement with goals of treatment. The evident tasks involved in achieving any *such* state of affairs are obviously staggering; if not frightening, they are still inescapable. To begin with, however, we may be content that at least their recognition—as well as intelligent efforts toward fulfilling them, however halting at first—are valuable additions to the therapeutic nature of the hospital's social structure.

The logic of this approach is that there must be a rather basic and accepted philosophy of treatment. The presence of such a factor in the hospital promotes a consistency of effort. Something of this nature, at least in part, may account for the fact that patients will tend to get well in treatment programs that differ radically from each other in other respects. The overall acceptance of an "approach" to treatment and the subsequent consistency of effort may then be factors which promote healthy changes in patients. If so, we would tend to look upon them as essential ingredients of the psychotherapeutic community.

The presence and exploration of differences of opinion is a healthy aspect of any community. It may be soundly argued, therefore, that common acceptance of a basic philosophy is antitherapeutic. Room for difference of opinions and their exploration must be maintained. However, while agreement that there may be disagreement is good, there must be maintained some knowledge of limits beyond which disagreement at any single time is considered antitherapeutic. The determination of these limits in a therapeutic community would seem best left in the hands of those most skilled in and most responsible for the treatment of the patient.

The medical "team approach" to the treatment of patients in a hospital would seem consistent with much of the above and therefore a logical feature of the therapeutic community. It may be debatable whether the medical staff should be "open" or "closed." However, in either event, to be a therapeutic factor as such, among themselves the medical team must have ample communication leading to mutual understanding and consistent agreement about broad treatment policies for all the patients, as well as treatment procedures for the individual patient for whom they also bear responsibility as a group. It would seem a sine qua non of the psychotherapeutic community that both chief responsibility and leadership for all aspects of the hospital be in the hands of the medical staff. This, too, would point up the need for unity among them, and consistency of approach on their part, for these promote the structured atmosphere so supportive and important to the patient's progress. The psychiatrist possesses the deepest understanding of the patient and is most aware of the extent to which daily decisions will affect the patient singly and as a group. In submitting himself to the consensus of "the team," he minimizes the chance that he will make antitherapeutic decisions.

The successful use of the team approach requires, among other things, that all avenues of communication finally lead to the medical staff and ultimately emanate from it. In addition, a high degree of emotional and temporal investment by the doctors in the therapeutic program is indispensable to success. Communication with the individual patient on the one-to-one office level only is hardly adequate. The psychiatrist must meet the patient as an individual and in groups on as many levels as possible and in as many different contexts and situations as possible.

Values and value systems are social factors in the therapeutic community. In the hospital treatment of psychiatric illnesses it is the impaired judgment of the patient which causes as much hardship for himself and others as any other feature of his illness. He is led to proclaim his uniqueness in various ways and will brook no limitation of his personal sovereignty. Usually he insists that his judgment be above question in even the most minor matters and that his values, no matter how whimsical, are absolute. As often as not it has been his extremely poor social judgment plus his adamant attitudes which have made him such a trial to himself and society as to require his hospitalization. Invariably, it would seem, he lives by a curiously individualistic system of values that serves only to perpetuate his social isolation.

The extent to which we are successful in helping the patient to choose a value system that is, in the main but not absolutely consonant with that of his community, is the measure of our therapeutic effectiveness. How to implement restrictive or corrective measures when we are required to do so without finding ourselves in a harsh and censorious role and without stirring up unmanageable antitherapeutic reaction is the technique we must perforce study. As the healthiest and most knowledgeable segment of the hospital community, the medical team will be responsible more than anyone else for defining the healthy limits of feeling, thought, and action, as well as the general goals and aims of the community. It will afford the patient the opportunity of committing himself to the attainment of good social judgment by helping him see that he will ultimately benefit in terms of improved mental health. What we have in mind is essentially a *learning process* for the patients as individuals and groups. The discovery and utilization of those conditions which are optimal for such learning by such patients is the main business of the therapeutic community. Our purpose is to expose our patient to social forces which will demonstrate to him a need as well as a clear choice to modify his aberrant value systems along healthier lines, thus enabling psychotic isolation and estrangement to give way to healthy integration into the immediate hospital community, and eventually into society at large.

Our observations indicate that insight and judgment improve in group interplay which considers and is guided by value judgments. It would be a sterile community indeed which was devoid of such interplay. It is a healthy one which can allow for such interplay in fair, objective, and constructive ways. The degree of understanding of each other with respect to their individual values and the coordination of these into viable social value systems is in large part determined by the quality of the communication which exists within this community of persons. The psychiatric hospital is often the very first significant opportunity afforded to the emotionally isolated individual for consensual validation of his values.

The therapeutic community, therefore, among other social factors, has to have a value system that is relatively acceptable to the medical team. This system is consciously exercised in opposition to the sick value system of the patient as an individual and the patients as groups. We act consciously in having the patient question his sick system of values and accepting ours instead. We do not impose it on him, but rather help him to make the positive step toward accepting a system which is more rationally geared to the fulfillment of his healthy human needs than was his own. It has been our observation that, as a general rule, to the extent we are successful in accomplishing this, the patient is successful in integrating himself into the hospital community, and that this sequence of events is usually attended by the amelioration of symptoms and the visible evidence of improved health.

Once we have recognized and accepted the role of social factors in the etiology and therapy of emotional illness, we are awed by the magnitude of the task that lies before us in the implementation of any system for the study and treatment of such illness. The investment of human resources, which we have intimated is necessary, is enormous. This fact alone may account in large measure for what we have recognized as a tendency to turn away from the development and perfection of our hospitals as psychotherapeutic communities. We are forced to turn towards what is expedient and away from what is truly therapeutic. The greatest danger, of course, is that in so doing we may confuse one with the other, expedience with scientific truth.

But we believe that what has never been done can be done. We look to the future in which the mental hospital is far from today's traditional concept of a hospital. It is a community of people not greatly unlike any other community of people in its physical aspects, though fundamentally different in its other aspects. We foresee that this hospital community will be, in addition, a social laboratory where the functional nature of man will be under as close a scrutiny as has been his physical and physiological nature in the past. We can foresee that one day the activities of patients in our hospital community will be broadened to include such categories of essentially human behavior as the full range of productive work and play, not merely the simulated activities which we see, for example, in traditional occupational therapy.

Our own experience suggests that as we learn more, introducing a bit at a time, we may eventually duplicate within the therapeutic hospital environment the greater part, if not the whole spectrum, of normal human social activity.

REFERENCES

1. Stanton, A. H., and M. D. Schwartz. *The mental hospital.* New York: Basic Books, 1954.

2. Caudill, W. *The psychiatric hospital as a small society.* Cambridge, Mass.: Harvard Univ. Press, 1958.

3. Cohen, R. A. "The hospital as a therapeutic instrument." *Psychiatry,* 2:29 (1958).

4. Schwartz, M., and C. G. Schwartz. "Considerations in determining a model for the mental hospital." *American Journal of Psychiatry,* 116:435 (1959).

5. Gralnick, A. "Inpatient psychoanalytic psychotherapy of schizophrenia." *Psychoanalysis and Human Values.* vol. 3, pg. 286. New York: Grune & Stratton, 1960.

6. Rabiner, Edwin *et al.* "The therapeutic community as an insight catalyst." *American Journal of Psychotherapy,* 18:2:244–58 (April 1964).

7. Opler, M. K. "Entities and organization in individual and group behavior." *Group Psychotherapy,* 9:4 (December 1956).

8. Jones, M. *The therapeutic community.* New York: Basic Books, 1953.

9. Krasner, L. "The therapist as a social reinforcement machine." *Research in Psychotherapy,* vol. 2.

10. Silverberg, J. W. *et al. The implementation of psychoanalytic concepts in hospital practice, science, and psychoanalysis,* vol. 3, 7. pg. 280. New York: Grune & Stratton, 1964.

Chapter 3
The Humanizing Influence of the Psychiatric Hospital

in collaboration with Frank G. D'Elia, M.D.

After an initial spurt of enthusiasm at the prospect of participating on this panel, I must confess to an ensuing difficult period of soul-searching and malaise. As the program committee and I originally worked out the title for my portion of the program, namely, "The Humanizing Influence of the Psychiatric Hospital," I believed the subject matter much to my liking, what with our hospital's emphasis on the therapeutic community and the study of interpersonal relationships. However, it soon became apparent that there was a big difference between returning the sick patient to his previous "normal" state and having a "humanizing" influence upon him. It began to appear that I had assumed more than that for which I had bargained, and I must confess to frequent bouts of regret at having agreed to tackle the subject at all.

As a psychiatrist given to a certain amount of introspection, I soon perceived the first part of my work cut out for me, namely, to explore my misgivings. Naturally, too, I wondered how my fellow panelists were faring, and whether they, also, were sharing the same doubts. Were the same questions occurring to them? Were they too thinking they had bitten off more than they could chew? Did they also believe that this panel was going to encounter a lot of trouble and had gotten hold of a tiger by the tail? Holding a tiger by the tail was one thing, but turning tail was quite another, and, as you can see, I decided to persevere, but

25

only with the help of a colleague member of our staff, Frank D'Elia, who coauthors this article.

It would seem in order, then, for us first to share with you the substance of our doubts and introspective efforts. All psychiatrists have their theory as to what causes mental illness, and they have some idea about how to proceed to remedy their patients' illness. However, they have differing ideas as to the roots of mental disorder. They differ even more about how scientifically to determine the cause of mental, let alone "emotional," malfunction. They may at times be vehement in their differences about the actual treatment of the mentally ill. More to the point, however, if psychiatrists are in disagreement about the cause and treatment of the subject of their endeavors, they are even more so about their opinions on the "normal" state of mental health. It is fair to say that the overwhelming portion of the efforts of psychiatrists is given over to a study of mental disorders. Very little time, and that only in more recent years, is given to a consideration of what is the normal state of mental health and how it is attained.

As our soul-searching continued we came to see a little more clearly what our "hang-up" was. We had been confusing "human" with "normal" and thinking of these terms synonymously. To think of our efforts as returning one's patient to a state of normality was one thing, and difficult enough, considering that what was "normal" was certainly debatable, and, how to achieve it was certainly controversial. However, to "humanize"—that is, make one's patient "human"—was certainly a horse of another color. The question, then, was, how did we get into that area in the first place and did we have any business in it in the second place—whether in a public or private hospital? If our main business to date had been freeing a patient of sick symptoms and calling the residue the "normal" state of mind (and that ploy had been difficult enough and not getting us any too far), where, then, would this tack lead us?

This kind of thinking surely led to what appeared to be some further serious reflection. Was the consideration of what was "human" and "humanizing" really the province of the psychiatrist? While most people continue to believe that the study and treatment of the mentally ill is still the concern of the psychiatrist and that therefore the study and determination of what is "normal" mentally is also his, we need to be mindful that increasingly voices, some of them quite shrill, are beginning to question even this. What, then, would be our fate if we began to get into the more controversial area of what is "human" and "humanizing"?

In some respects the dilemma posed and developed here has had a logical evolution. As psychiatrists we have somehow wandered to it ourselves, and it is of our own making, or we have been led there by others willy-nilly—either passive and unconscious dupes or willing slaves to the social and political pressures of our times. Particularly psychoanalysts, and psychiatrists as their jealous first cousins, have permitted society to assign to them certain powers of understanding, and to a certain extent—through their study of sick individuals—have attributed to themselves certain omniscient powers of understanding, not merely of the individual, but also of groups of people, classes of society, sections of the world, crime waves, religious and political movements, and all manner of social, political, and military upheaval.

We ourselves have always objected to the fact that psychiatrists often pose as experts or are taken as experts in any area other than that for which they have been trained. We have regretted such efforts as doing them a disservice as psychiatrists and doing an injury to psychiatry as a medical specialty. We have held to the belief that psychiatry and psychoanalysis are medical specialties to be practiced only by medical men and women for one main reason, to wit, that they exclusively are given a type of clinical experience and training—over and above necessary training in the basic sciences and anatomy and physiology, etc.—which is the key ingredient in the adequate observation, understanding, and treatment of the mentally ill. We have, therefore, taken exception to the excursions of some of our colleagues, leaning on their reputations and expertise as psychiatrists, into the realms of politics, religion, philosophy, sociology, and anthropology, among others. This does not mean that we believe psychiatrists should not take stands on the burning issues of our times. They should! But only as individuals who do not permit their deserved reputations as psychiatrists to be used to anoint them as experts in these other areas.

With this as the background of our thinking, how could we find it palatable to accept this assignment? Our conclusion was that we could only do so as clinicians, not as philosophers or sociologists. If we could find the clinical path to what humanizes the patient, if we could at least convey that this alone was the direction for psychiatry to take, or if we could find how clinically to assist the patient himself to find the route, or if we could show that our clinical management of the patient helps him see the need to acquire certain human qualities and thereby pursue their development—then we ourselves could see a consistency between our beliefs and the pursuit of the subject matter.

At High Point we have emphasized the continuing improvement of the hospital entity as a "human" instrument, and have concentrated on understanding and improving our responses to mental illness so that they might be therapeutic. We have considered the motivations and techniques involved in such a goal as essentially human, that the humanizing effect is on the practitioner as well as on the patient. The latter must perforce incorporate a large amount of the essential humanity of the psychiatrist because of the very structure of the relationship. It is deeper and designed both to influence the way in which the patient thinks, feels, and acts, and to bring him into accord with certain clinically selected thoughts and feelings of the psychiatrist.

We accept patients because we know that we can offer them significant help toward becoming well. Our hospital structure and our own responses to illness have been specialized to be therapeutic. This is in contrast to the families of patients and to the societal groups in which they moved. These are usually panicked and confused by the phenomenon of mental illness, and respond in a manner which usually compounds the patient's difficulties. We, then, have become specialized by a combination of clinical experience and humanistic theory which, in turn, is its fruit.

We had long accepted the importance of including certain clinically selected values in the treatment process by making them known to patients. We knew we had not been preaching at our patients and that any such approach was neither clinical nor fruitful. As we deliberated in this preliminary fashion we sensed that our clinical program had been exercising a humanizing influence and that we could accept the topic as a challenge to clarify these elements in our program and to explore further ways in which any program could go about exerting a humanizing influence on its patients.

Anyone undertaking to influence the human qualities of a patient in a hospital setting must have and know his own concepts of what is "human"—as opposed to "normal"—and develop clinical techniques of conveying them to the awareness of patients. His techniques must extend to the point that permits patients to aspire to and acquire them if they so wish. At the least, these treatment techniques should communicate to the patient the importance of human qualities to the state of his mental health and thereby inspire in him the desire and ability to recognize and develop in himself these very qualities. Further, these techniques should convey to the patient the knowledge that exercising a humanizing influence on another is, in itself, humanizing and productive of mental health. It is no secret to us, of course, that this approach constitutes a part of our own value system, but by the same token, it has been gleaned from our clinical experience in the treatment of the mentally ill.

While all of us are human beings, we tend to grade ourselves as more or less "human," depending on our own individual scale of values. Certain of us seem to be invested with more "human" qualities than others and surpass others in being "human" in their relationships. Some are kinder, more charitable, more understanding, more forgiving, more altruistic, more sensitive, and so on. Generally, then, we seem to think of the more "human" person as being the more positive in his relations with his fellow man. We may differ in the list of such qualities we include and in the degree to which we think they should exist in a person, but we generally concede that the possession of such qualities is what sets one apart as more or less human. Further, we agree that the person who is, contrariwise, cruel, sadistic, selfish, insensitive, etc., is the less "human."

Should psychiatrists in a hospital setting, then, attempt to germinate in patients such qualities where they may be lacking

or develop them further where they may be minimal in degree? If
the answer is in the affirmative, such psychiatrists must defend
the thesis that "humanity" minimizes mental illness. Not an
easy thesis to defend! Is, then, the way back to mental health
through the development of human qualities and the practice of
humanity? Not an easy question to answer, let alone justify!
This tack, then, again forces the question: Is this the realm of
psychiatry or religion? Of psychiatry as a medical specialty or as
a social discipline? Of psychiatry—or philosophy?

We ourselves are not now prepared to respond fully to any of
these questions. Instead, at this juncture, we are tempted to ask
even more to which psychiatrists must address themselves if
they enter this particular arena. From whence come these qualities which determine the degree of our humanity? Why do they
vary so in us? Are they genetically determined? If socially
determined, why are the positive, as well as the negative, human
qualities found in all strata of society? And why in this society,
which we boast to be the most highly developed, are the negative human qualities so increasingly rampant, let alone the mental disorders so prevalent? And is there any relationship between
these facts? What of hunger and starving children in our affluent
society? What of the credibility gap? What of war? What of all
sorts of human want and degradation in the face of the most
exalted and sublime? And what of the effect of such inconsistencies on the psychology of all of us? The critical point we would
make here is that the grossly negative aspects of our society
must also have a devastating emotional effect on those who do
not directly suffer these miseries because their very existence is
in such sharp conflict with the teachings and values upon which
all of us rest our stability and strength.

And what compels psychiatrists, whose sole claim is that of
clinicians and psychiatric hospital administrators, to ask such
pregnant questions? Only the nature of the subject matter facing
us! These queries are unavoidable! While we can attempt
their answer, we do not believe this is the forum for them. Yet
the dilemma for us as hospital psychiatrists remains. We may
not be able to adequately answer these questions, but we certainly can study and point up the devastating effect their overtones have on the mental health of all human beings.

We have learned from our own clinical experience that the study and practice of "human" relationships within a hospital setting helps lead to mental health in patients. Further, such study of both the patient and professional staff leads to an awareness of the presence or absence of, and the true degree of their respective, human qualities. Under the proper conditions of communication there may actually occur an enhancement of such qualities. The clinical program interested in the human development of its participants engages in a close study of the reality of its setting. It seeks full awareness of the true and real role of everyone in the environment. In this process each is motivated to clarify what is expected of him as a human being in his goal-directed activity, namely, the fulfillment of his respective responsibilities in the most effective manner. Beyond awareness of what is expected of him, this type of social structure promotes in each an acceptance of the obligations of his assigned role and a recognition that their fulfillment leads to the disappearance of symptoms and the emergence and improvement of human qualities. Human relationships are studied not merely so each may learn what he is like and how he may function more effectively, but how he may more rationally (humanly) fulfill his task in the hospital. All ultimately recognize their significance in the fulfillment of the hospital's real purpose, namely, the adequate care and treatment of the patient, the training and development of its professional staff, and the general objective of a job well done by and for everybody.

We would draw a distinction between our emphasis and the "humanitarian" approach that favors the open door, freedom, kindness, sympathy, and love as the tools of treatment. These alone are not enough and may be misapplied to inadvertently injure rather than help if used without plan and technical clinical design or psychiatric awareness of the patient's malady. All of us know that, quite to the contrary, firmness, restraint, structured control, frustration, and denial are often more helpful.

We recognize that thus far we have but skimmed the surface and left rather untouched the actual techniques and detailed description of the hospital's social structure necessary for it to exercise a humanizing influence. Time does not permit even an outline of the design of the needed social relationships, the complex communication system, ,and the network of human interrelationships, yet they are the very elements which compel study and awareness of one's self as a "human" being, and further, indicate the necessity for and direction of the "human" change. Broadly speaking, however, the clinical technique is in the manner of relating to, living with, and dealing with the patient in the social structure of the hospital of which we speak. As a matter of fact, these very elements constitute the structure. This hospital is a society, a social setting, a culture with established ways of living, mores, and value systems. It has a past, a current life, and a direction into the future. It is a living process, not a static environment in which techniques of treatment are somehow carried out apart from this process.

It is clear that what we express is a far cry from the ordinary medical model which seeks merely to erase symptoms and return the patient to the premorbid state. Such a model is unrelated to any humanizing influence. In order to "humanize" the patient we must have a particular type of human relationship with him. Insight is not enough, apart from the special human aspects of our relationship with the patient which aims to bridge the chasm which separates him from others. The problems implicit in this approach, of course, have been the subject matter of this article.

The updated treatment model we favor involves much more than the alleviation of symptoms by physical means in a brief hospital stay. We are probably suggesting here the essence of the therapeutic community concept. We are speaking of a consciously designed social structure, clinical in its work of dealing with an illness accepted as medical, whose proponents are aware that they employ techniques of treatment which must touch the patient's humanity if his symptoms are to be alleviated. This, in a way, expresses the core of the concept of the psychiatric hospital as a therapeutic instrument.

Chapter 4
"Administration" as Therapy of the Inpatient's Family

in collaboration with Frank G. D'Elia, M.D.

One cannot overemphasize the belief that the hospital's management of the family of an inpatient should be seen as a therapeutic task. The underlying concept is that "the hospital" is an administrative unit, that is, a social exchange system of people, and that it may affect the family therapeutically. In other words, just as a hospital may coordinate its personnel to affect the direction of a patient's life, so it may conduct its affairs to influence some change in the family's life style. Its relationship to family members will be sufficiently intense in enough vital areas to affect their orientation and reaction patterns. The "hospital" may be consciously designed to relate to the family so as to educate it in new ways of thinking and viewing family relationships. Ordinarily a family mistakenly looks upon administration as the "business" end of the hospitalization which is devoid of human emotion. Sad to say, many psychiatrists think similarly and convey such misconceptions to families. This, however, will not be true if "administration" is intimately related to the treatment team and its relationship to the family integrated with the therapeutic approach to the patient. This requires close involvement of the chief psychiatrist in a leadership role in both administration and the therapeutic program. He is a liaison agent between the two and should view "administration" and "therapy" as two sides of the same coin. The whole concept involves even more, namely, accepting knowledgeable "administration" as

33

therapy, since it involves human transactions. Admittedly, implementation of these concepts is most difficult.

Family therapy came upon the psychiatric scene fairly recently with a burst of enthusiasm and a large measure of hope. It quickly acquired adherents and became entrenched as attempts were made to define its limits and techniques. The alacrity with which family therapy was adopted is comprehensible in the light of our relative inadequacy in psychiatry. However, instead of there having arisen some uniform understanding of family pathology, some common theory about family dynamics, or some consistent technique of family therapy, quite the reverse has occurred. In every respect there are widely divergent opinions within a specific culture, let alone cross-culturally. As Ackerman stated, "The most striking feature of our field today is the emergence of a bewildering array of diverse forms of family treatment. Each therapist seems to be doing his own thing."[1] This very idea we are attempting to delineate and implement is but an example of one "doing his own thing." If it needs "justification," it is self-evident in the light of our deficiencies in dealing with the mentally ill and their families. Our need to learn and advance our methods is plain.

It is interesting that prior to the advent of family therapy, only a few studies of families had been made. The prominent ones traced the presence of mental illness in families through several generations and had special interest from the genetic standpoint. A family study one of us had the privilege of making in the early 1940s encouraged a different emphasis. In a paper entitled, "The Carrington Family: A Psychiatric and Social Study Illustrating the Psychosis of Association or Folie à Deux,"[2] an attempt was made to show that the pathology of a mother could affect her children and husband, that pathology could then exist in each member of a family unit, and that social factors could promote family psychopathology. This study was done in conjunction with another on folie à deux[3] (or, as it was called then, "psychosis of association"), a pathological condition long known as one in which one sick person could affect or "infect" another with his disease process.

After some years of state hospital experience associated with analytic training, followed by psychoanalytic practice solely devoted to the intrapsychic and interpersonal study and treatment of the individual, there followed the founding by one of us in 1951 of a psychiatric hospital devoted to psychoanalytically oriented psychotherapy of the psychoses. This background is given to show that, given a particular type of hospital experience with such a background of training, one would naturally pioneer in the field of family therapy with the inpatient concurrently with the efforts being made at family therapy in office practice.

By tradition, the psychoanalyst refrained from seeing family members of his ambulatory patient because of the theoretical premises underlying his work. The nonanalytic psychiatrist leaned heavily on the physiological therapies so that his contact with family members was relatively superficial, certainly not one resembling an intimate or therapeutic nature. The state hospital psychiatrist was too burdened to see family members, so that by tradition the social worker substituted for him and maintained other than a therapeutic relation to the family. Until recently the private hospital was certainly influenced by state hospital tradition if it emphasized organic therapy and by psychoanalytic theory if it emphasized psychotherapy and milieu therapy. In either case, it employed social workers to maintain contact with the family.

This, then, was the situation when High Point Hospital was begun in 1951 and was facing organizational problems. In keeping with prevailing tradition, we should have employed social workers to deal with families, particularly since the hospital was originally designed to render psychoanalytic psychotherapy. Psychiatrists, therefore, would have been free to maintain their special therapeutic relationship with the patient "untainted" by contact with the family. Had this been done we might yet be functioning, as do most hospitals, with social workers maintaining primary contact with the patient's family.

However, we strayed from tradition, because in the earliest years of High Point Hospital, budgetary limitations made the employment of social workers impossible. Consequently, the therapist had to deal with the relatives of patients. Of course, this exposure initiated us into what was then the new field of family therapy and ultimately to "our own thing." Subsequently, we read our first formal paper on family therapy in the hospital setting in 1957[4] and have followed it with others in the succeeding years.

Initially we made many observations, some of which bear repeating here. We found many family members genuinely interested in the patient; that if they were hostile, they were also loving; that many were sympathetic to our therapeutic problems as well as being negatively inclined toward us; that some were trusting of us though many were suspicious; and that many were frightened, anxious, angry, frustrated, ignorant of the patient's psychopathology, guilt-ridden, truly suffering human beings. We found that they had control over the patient and us through the "power of the purse," that they could and would wield it by removing the patient from our care for any number of reasons. We found that most were suspicious of and angry at the psychiatrist who had previously treated the patient. They complained that he had refused to see them despite their desire to see him. They, therefore, had had no chance to tell him what had really been occurring with the patient. Now the patient was in the hospital, and "it was the doctor's fault"! Further, the psychiatrist had not told them how serious things were; "unaccountably" and unexpectedly the patient had attempted to commit suicide. Perhaps they could have prevented it. Now, suddenly, he was in the hospital. And what did we hospital psychiatrists think of such colleagues? Did they, therefore, now have any reason to trust us? How would we be treating them?

Here, then, was "the hospital"—not the therapist as an isolate—faced with a role and policy it had to assume "administratively" in reaction to this common fashion in which the family related to it. The family's attitudes were critically important to the therapeutic result. Naturally, hospital response called for the utmost circumspection with respect to the family's feelings, the referring psychiatrist and professional ethics, as well as tolerance for the differing techniques of psychotherapy. They were essential to the patient's welfare. We knew the latter depended on a close understanding and trust between the family and the hospital, as well as between the patient and his family. An administrative policy had to be evolved to insure all of the above through thorough education and indoctrination. Variation from such policy could be catastrophic to the therapeutic process.

In retrospect we would say that family complaints were justified, that psychiatrists treated many of them grievously but in keeping with theory. At any rate, we ourselves quickly saw that the nature of our particular hospital practice with the psychotic patient and the way we related to his family were unique. Ackerman says that family therapy arose from the experience of psychiatrists in treating children rather than schizophrenics.[5] Unfortunately, this was true in office practice, but it might just as well have arisen from the ambulatory treatment of the schizophrenic. In our experience, family therapy seemed inevitable to our early specialized hospital program. Today, any hospital that wishes to do better with its patients should engage in such therapy, no matter what its principal emphasis, and, as an administrative unit, seek to affect the family.

We soon found that if we were to work effectively with our patients, let alone have a lengthy opportunity to treat them, we had to work with their families. For the reasons already mentioned, we developed a rapport with them. Since we lived closely and worked intensively with our patients on a 24-hour basis, we had an additional reason for being sympathetic with the family. All of us could see and experience with patients exactly what relatives had had to tolerate and sometimes suffer. We soon came to avoid rationalizing that any of our unhealthy reaction to patients was merely "countertransference," while that of the family was "psychopathology" (in referring here to *we,* the authors mean all of the administrative and professional staff as a team). We found that we sorely needed and had to win the understanding and cooperation of the family if we were to be successful, and the families discovered that they needed ours.

We often observed that individual relatives were mature and that families, as such, could be quite healthy despite a psychotic member. We found that some families had seemed disturbed prior to the patient's hospitalization, but that they stabilized readily once the patient was removed. Accordingly, we were not loathe to think of the patient as the primarily sick one. Out of ignorance and helplessness the family appeared pathological only as it tried its best to cope with its sick member. We began to believe that the primary patient, if sick enough, could very well make for a sick family. At the moment, contrary to many students of the subject, we doubt the idea that a sick family necessarily makes the sick member or that if you find a sick individual you have found a sick family. We would just as soon believe that if you find a sick family you have found a sick culture in which it has been living. A family, too, is not "an island unto itself"; it needs to be drawn into therapy by the hospital.

The fact that one member is hospitalized makes it evident that the family in question can no longer live as a unit at home. The patient himself is now under 24-hour observation and seen "in action" as he "lives out" and "acts out" his usual patterns of behavior. At the same time, however, the family members may also be seen "in action" through the many facets of their relationship to "the hospital." For instance, how the family handles the hospital's many rules and regulations is significant and revealing. What is the family's "personality" and what are its various attitudes? Is it cooperative and understanding or suspicious and insensitive? Does it demonstrate real or casual interest in the patient? Does it pay its bills on time? Is it fault-finding with the hospital's administrative practices? Does it trust the patient's therapist or blame him for every sign of the patient's regression? Does it displace its hostility and become critical of "administrative authority" when the patient shows signs of improvement? Does it enter family therapy willingly when it is suggested? Does it uniformly blame the patient or assume a share of responsibility for the family's plight? These questions give some clues to understanding family dynamics and transactional techniques which need to be learned in order to relate successfully to families.

The hospital presses and pressures the family in many practical ways. Its demands interfere with and shake the family's daily routine and equilibrium. It is a threat in that it may elicit the family's innermost secrets and expose it to shame and stigma. A good communication system enables the hospital which involves the families to see them in "living action" much more so than the office practitioner of family therapy, for the family members are reacting to many more people than the patient and his therapist and in many more emotionally laden situations. The hospital may be regarded as a living organism, a society with its own laws and value systems, all of which are brought to bear on the family. The family has its own systems and values, which inevitably clash with those of the hospital. Naturally, the hospital needs to be more stable and rational in its system if it is to help the patient and his family. Its aim is to bring its patients (the selected patient and the family) into harmony with its own system. The hospital must also be flexible and bring itself into accommodation with its patients at appropriate times.

The essence of family therapy is that the patient be seen in the context of the family if he is to be adequately understood and treated. By the same token, it would seem that the family needs to be seen in the wider context of the greater culture if it itself is to be better understood and treated. This, of course, brings us into the area of social psychiatry and the manifold attendant problems it presents us as psychiatrists in our respective cultures. It seems to us, at any rate, that in the proper hospital setting, one has a golden opportunity to treat the family in its broader social context. The office practitioner who treats a family deals with a wider context than when he treats the single patient but a lesser social context than that of the hospital psychiatrist treating the family. The social system of the hospital is much more demanding of both the patient and the family. It is a much more complex and complicated social system. For example, it has removed the patient from the family, it houses and cares for him entirely, and it is responsible for his very being, not just his interpersonal life. In this respect, its responsibilities are much greater. Where such a condition prevails, the social pressures are more comprehensive, and the family is affected more thoroughly.

In office practice there are numerous forms of family therapy, a fact that can be understood only in terms of the multivaried nature of the psychiatrist's training, life experience, personality, and cultural background, let alone the heritage and pathology of the family he is treating. The forms family therapy takes in hospital practice, aside from the fact that it is not commonly done in hospitals, may be explained similarly. Logic suggests that if our own thinking about the form of family therapy is to be understood, the hospital program itself should be described and its theoretical orientation understood, for, after all, it is the wider social system in which the patient and his family are involved.

Our hospital is a 45-bed institution devoted to psychoanalytically oriented psychotherapy. It has a "closed staff" of seven full-time psychiatrists who work as a team in treating its 40 patients. Incidentally, these therapists come to us from various parts of the world and therefore represent different cultures, but successfully treat patients from our particular culture. Though each patient is given three individual therapeutic sessions a week, most decisions about him are made by team consensus. There is a highly developed therapeutic milieu, and the nursing staff is actively engaged with the doctors in observing and decision-making concerning the patients. The hospital also has a sophisticated communications system and many staff conferences in which the patients' treatment is constantly reviewed. Electroshock is not used, although psychotropic drugs are. Elderly and organic cases are excluded, as are acute alcoholics; adolescents are often in the majority, and are treated along with adults. Patient stays average six months, and the bulk of patients suffer from some form of schizophrenia.

Basically, we believe that a patient's illness arises from unhealthy living conditions and relationships, that the process can be arrested and reversed in a relatively healthy environment. We believe that a psychiatric hospital may be that kind of a rational environment. We believe, further, that as a group of people, we bring more than our technical knowledge to bear on patients and families, namely, our system of values. We believe that it takes more than insight into a patient's intrapsychic life to effect change in him and that it is the current effect of the total living process of the hospital which affects the patient. Similarly, we believe that the hospital's total process affects the family therapeutically. This is to say, the "management" of the family assists its therapy.

Following our early, primitive efforts to treat families— sympathizing with them and gaining their understanding, educating them, gaining their cooperation, supporting them, relieving them of their anxiety and guilt feelings—we embarked on more formal methods of family therapy. When timely, a therapist saw a patient regularly, together with one or more significant members of the family. Sometimes the patient's therapist saw family members separately. If this was not feasible, another member of the staff saw the family in collaborative therapy. Soon we found ourselves using the variations of family therapy familiar to office practitioners and with more or less the same aim: that all gain insight, so that eventually they could live together more harmoniously. In this stage of the development of family therapy in our facility, the hospital served as the reasonable environment in which the therapist, patient, and family could meet, but still be rather divorced from the hospital as such. It was as though the hospital, as an organization of interested people, played no role and had nothing to offer this particular therapeutic process in our total treatment program. Yet this state of affairs was inconsistent with our general thinking that the total hospital process played an important part in the therapy, that no part was separable from the others. With the passage of time, this contradiction increasingly became evident.

As we gave this some thought, certain major ideas came to the fore. Family therapy had been designed to help a family's members gain insight into themselves as individuals and as a group so that they could more easily solve the problems they had in living together. In the process the therapist observed how they behaved and made interpretations intended to alter such behavior and associated feelings. Our hospital was very small, and its many professionals, both medical and administrative, were so intimately involved with the patient—and the family— that they could be considered extensions of the family. Additionally, the family members were drawn into intimate relationship with our total staff and were under close observation, so that what and how they did or said things could be easily seen and heard, interpreted for them on the spot, or reported to the medical staff and patient's therapist, to be used for interpretation in the more formal family sessions.

An example may help clarify how a member of a family demonstrates his psychopathology in relation to the hospital and how it, in turn, may deal with him therapeutically. When a father brings his son to the hospital for care, he signs an obligation agreement and thereby assumes the responsibility to meet the fees in a prescribed manner in return for professional and other services the hospital promises to render. The parent then reveals himself when he begins to neglect this responsibility, quarrels about insignificant parts of the bills, tells the patient's therapist that he trusts him but not the hospital, and yet maintains his son in the hospital with the full expectation that it will fulfill its services to the patient. He thus tries to divorce himself, his son, and the therapist from the hospital and rationalizes his delinquency and thoughtlessness, if not hostility, toward his son as demonstrated by this behavior toward those who are caring for his supposed loved one. The hospital, in turn, may manage the parent in several ways. Administration may report the matter to the patient's therapist for him to deal with either individually with the parent or in a family session. Or administration may refuse to extend credit to the patient so that he, in turn, must face it out with the parent. On the other hand, it may tell the parent or turn to the medical director and tell him that the hospital will no longer treat the patient in the face of the parent's irresponsibility, thus forcing the logic of the latter's behavior upon his consciousness. This course may compel him to raise the matter with the patient's therapist in the family sessions.

The hospital conveys to the relative that its ultimate success with the patient depends on three factors—the patient, the hospital, and the family. The more there is understanding, mutuality of goal, and harmony between them, the better the chance of a therapeutic success. The hospital is always striving to do its part, but in many ways, the patient will manipulate and resist therapy. The family, then, is very important to the treatment process and must work closely with the hospital. If it flouts the hospital's culture, it is not likely that the hospital can get the patient to do better. If it falls prey to the patient's manipulations and then covertly or overtly fights the hospital, the latter has both the family and patient to deal with—a severe handicap to its efforts. More than an educative process is involved here, because the hospital is dealing with the personality of the relative and his way of relating to both the patient and those caring for him. The hospital's management (administrative) efforts are directed toward giving the relative insight and altering his behavior. These are essential aspects of the therapeutic process.

Our thesis, then, is that management—or administration—and therapy are two sides of the same coin. In a hospital setting each has elements of the other, and they are inseparable. This is true of the program's relation to both the patient and the family. The behavior and emotional reactions of the staff affect the patient, just as his affect them. Thus when a patient causes staff to become overanxious or too apprehensive, they will have an adverse effect on him, and a vicious cycle will be maintained. Accordingly, they will need reassurance, but he will need medication, if only to minimize their adverse reactions. Similarly, the family and hospital may become involved in an unhealthy posture which needs remedial management or therapeutic methods. The methods of therapy may vary from family counseling and education to manipulation and experiential therapy, with the emphasis on confrontation. These may be carried on by the individual therapist or by the administrative arm of the hospital.

The purpose of family therapy is to extend the family's limits of adequacy and its social horizons. It is important, therefore, to understand the traits and attitudes of families and their members, which are characteristic both of a culture and a class. Though they will vary widely, knowledge of them may lead to better understanding and treatment of the individual and the family as an aggregate. However, it is probably not within the psychiatrist's ken to master the vast store of knowledge involved. Also, this approach evolves from the psychoanalytic tradition and tends to confine the psychiatrist to the boundaries of the family itself. This restriction has already proven inadequate, and knowledgeable family therapists are already beginning to look to the wider concept of *society* to better understand and affect the family.

In this connection, then, it would seem advisable for the psychiatrist to gain some measure of knowledge of the broader social, political, and economic factors, as well as the human values of a culture which affect its people. This is the social approach which poses very special problems for psychiatry. It is the essence of our thinking in relation to the management of the family of the inpatient as a social unit, in relation to the hospital as a social organization. Just as there is no individual patient apart from his family and no family apart from its larger social matrix, so there is no administration distinct from its hospital's social structure and no hospital untouched by the larger society. All of these considerations (and more to be discovered) enter into the administrative therapy of the inpatient's family.

SUMMARY

We have advanced the thesis that an emotional impact on the inpatient's family is promoted through its management by "administration." The effect on the family may be therapeutic, or it may be the reverse. Accordingly, administrative personnel have a therapeutic task; they must relate to family with this well in mind. They are not merely the business part of the program, but are an integral part of the therapeutic team, working in close harmony with it. Under such conditions their transactions may contain the elements which promote healthy change. They may convey insight and compel alterations in family behavior through the very nature of the administrative process. In their administrative capacity, sophisticated personnel may educate and suggest. Importantly, they too convey the hospital's value system, which may clash with that of the family. The resolution of such conflict also is customarily therapeutic.

Our experience with families, the development of our concepts, and the rationale for our ideas and techniques has been described. The subject matter is an uncharted area with much potential and is worthy of further attention.

REFERENCES

1. Ackerman, N. W. "Family psychotherapy today." *Family Process,* 9:2 (June 1970).
2. Gralnick, A. "The Carrington family: a psychiatric and social study illustrating the psychosis of association or folie à deux." *Psychiatric Quarterly,* 17:294–326 (April 1943).
3. Gralnick, A. "Folie à deux: the psychosis of association." *Psychiatric Quarterly,* Part 1 (April 1942), Part 2 (July 1942).
4. Lefebvre, P., J. Atkins, J. Duckman, and A. Gralnick. "The role

of the relative in a psychotherapeutic program: anxiety problems and defensive reactions encountered.'' *Canadian Psychiatric Association Journal,* 3:3:110–18 (July 1958).

5. Ackerman, N. W. *The psychodynamics of family life.* New York: Basic Books, 1958.

Chapter 5
The Proprietary Psychiatric
Hospital: To Be or
Not to Be

The man or woman who elects to become a doctor starts a career of choice-making—what medical school, what location, what effort and for what return, what hospital for internship, what specialty and what hospital for it, where to practice, and finally, what branch of the specialty. Not that this finally ends the quest for answers; but we only stop at this point because we are directing our attention to the special field of the proprietary psychiatric hospital.

In thinking of his career in psychiatry today one needs first to reflect on the national scene as it is currently and promises to be in the foreseeable future. Among the significant conditions seriously affecting us are: the recently ended war; its effect upon the economy and the people's morale; the deep divisions of opinion which are polarizing the population relative to the war, and the civil and economic rights of minority groups; the generation gap and the disaffection of the young; the "drug and sexual revolution"; the rising incidence of hunger and crime; and the mounting threat of man's unrelenting assault upon his environment.

Important as all of these are, the developing psychiatrist will be most affected by the recent concept and rapidly accepted new value system, that the enjoyment of quality medical care is a "right" belonging to all. This has been quickly grasped by the mass of people who now demand its rapid implementation. Significant segments of our society are proceeding to satisfy this new set of values. In fact, most reasonable people now believe that national health insurance will be a reality by the time the present first-year resident completes his training.

The Group for the Advancement of Psychiatry has forcibly brought to our attention the serious dilemma of all psychiatric hospitals today. While we will restrict our concerns to the proprietary hospital, we should be aware of the G.A.P. paper which states, "This report is a protest against a current band-wagon movement exemplified by such slogans as: Keep patients out of psychiatric hospitals as much as you can; use the psychiatric ward of a general hospital instead of a mental hospital; the only good psychiatry is treatment in the community."[1] G.A.P. believes that the current emphasis threatens the existence of all psychiatric hospitals.

The proprietary psychiatric hospital conducts its program with two essential aims in mind: (1) that its patients will respond to appropriate therapy, and (2) that professional as well as financial profit will accrue to those who have invested their time, money, and skill to start or continue the facility. In this latter respect, it is no different from the vast majority of ventures in our free-enterprise system, including the private practice of medicine. Proprietary psychiatric hospitals have widely differing features. They vary in size (up to some 300 beds), may be "open-staffed" or "closed-staffed," and under the ownership of a single individual or a group of individuals. The owners may be psychiatrists or a combination of psychiatrists, laymen, and other physicians, or they may be only laymen. In most states, however, regardless of the nature of the proprietor, only a qualified psychiatrist may be issued the license to operate the program. This makes him personally liable for all that occurs under his direction. In some states, a corporation may be licensed to operate the institution, but for accreditation purposes, the person in charge of the treatment program will invariably be a qualified psychiatrist.

Some proprietary hospitals emphasize individual, group, and milieu therapy, alone or in combination with one or another form of physical therapy. Others emphasize the physical therapies alone, or in some loose combination with one or another form of nonphysical therapy. Some hospitals concentrate on the functionally ill, while others treat a significant proportion of organic illnesses. The age of the patients which the hospital admits varies, as does the proportion of each age group.

All proprietary hospitals concentrate primarily on the clinical treatment of the patient, while some give weight to research and residency training as well. Some prize pieces of research and pioneering therapeutic approaches have emanated from proprietary hospitals, and some of our great psychiatrists received their basic training in proprietary programs. Several presidents of the American Psychiatric Association, while in office, have had their chief affiliation with proprietary hospitals. This is true of both the current president and the upcoming president-elect.

Proprietary hospitals are found in both urban and suburban areas; most, however, are located in the well-populated sections of the nation. Some direct their main efforts to the long-term treatment of the chronic schizophrenic, though most seem to be responding to the current trend in psychiatry—that hospitalization be brief and the patient be returned quickly to the community. American history records that many of our finest nonprofit private and foundation hospitals started as proprietary programs. Most proprietary psychiatric hospitals are accredited by the Joint Commission on Accreditation of Hospitals.

Proprietary psychiatric hospitals are self-sustaining and may remain viable only as such. They are completely dependent upon their earned fees, and may not receive tax-free gifts of any kind. They may not receive research grants, fellowships, or residency training grants. Should they wish to expand or improve their programs, they may not receive Hill-Burton funds nor borrow money from the government under any conditions. They may resort to borrowing from banks or individuals only at current interest rates. Despite the crying need for psychiatric beds, there are numerous other difficulties which tend to hamper the initiation, growth, and even existence of the proprietary hospital. In this regard, however, there are some early signs of a contrary trend which will be touched upon later.

Proprietary psychiatric hospitals, as distinct from their fellow nonprofit private institutions, are subject to federal, state, and local school and real estate taxes. They receive no "breaks" or advantages from utilities, no "free services" from the community or "volunteer services," no matter what the extent of free professional time they may give the community in one form or another. Exceptions to this state of affairs are rare. They may not be part of a federally funded community mental health center. I have known patients compelled to enter state hospitals outside of their community because the local mental health board was forbidden to contract for bed space with a nearby proprietary hospital which could have cared for the patient in his own community. This situation exists despite the current emphasis that the patient is best treated in his own community.

Nevertheless, in the face of the above and contrary to common belief, fees in the best accredited, proprietary psychiatric hospitals are not higher, and in many cases are lower, than those in comparable private nonprofit, tax-free institutions. They compare most favorably even with the costs of the active treatment units of county and state hospitals. This would seem a state of affairs which requires very close study by responsible authorities. Fortunately, there are signs of such interest on the part of several states, as well as the federal government. Overall, one may wonder why and how the owners of proprietary psychiatric hospitals begin these enterprises, struggle to insure their survival, and in some instances actually achieve a position of eminence.

There is an aspect of hospital psychiatry of which one should be aware if one contemplates a career in this field. There seems to be a scale of evaluation—something resembling a hierarchy— of these institutions. The "scale" includes the quality as well as the prestige of the hospital. At the top is the private nonprofit, or foundation hospital, and then in descending order the state, federal, county and, finally, the proprietary psychiatric hospital. There are, of course, some exceptions to the rule; there are also some exceptions which "prove" the rule. It is likely that this "scale" has historical roots buried in the distant past, but I believe that there is no basis in fact for it. It is more likely that this outmoded method of measuring hospitals has as its base emotional biases. Having been the medical director of a proprietary hospital and having been exposed to the various matters I have mentioned, I am less than objective in this regard, colleagues have suggested.

The foregoing may well leave the young psychiatrist aghast and wary of the thought of entering the proprietary psychiatric hospital field. He may be quite puzzled, since this is being written by one who, in 1951, inaugurated a proprietary hospital and has been its medical director and proprietor ever since. However, there is every reason for serious consideration of the proprietary psychiatric hospital as a career. What has been written thus far is intended as the initial stage of an effort to present various aspects of the subject matter toward helping the young psychiatrist make an appropriate career choice.

The majority of proprietary psychiatric hospitals are members of the National Association of Private Psychiatric Hospitals. The Association is also comprised of many of the country's leading nonprofit and foundation hospitals. It plays a leading role in psychiatry, demands the highest standards for membership, promotes and guards the interest of psychiatric hospitals, and fosters the best treatment programs for patients. About 4,000 psychiatrists are associated with private hospitals on either a part- or full-time basis. The total membership of the Association is 131 hospitals, of which 73 are proprietary in nature. In round figures, the total bed capacity is about 19,000 beds, of which 6,500, about one-third, are in proprietary hospitals. However, of the total admissions of 87,000 per year, a majority of 48,000 were in the proprietary hospitals. Any reader who is interested in private hospital psychiatry as a career can communicate with the National Association of Private Psychiatric Hospitals, 353 Broad Avenue, Leonia, New Jersey 07605. To quote from the preface of its 1971 Directory: "The NAPPH is dedicated to helping all psychiatric facilities maintain quality care and high standards of treatment and conducts an extensive educational campaign through consultation services, conferences, national and regional meetings, seminars, publications and multi-media courses for this purpose. Its committees and task forces are committed to conduct studies in many areas to improve quality of performance. The NAPPH is an active participant in the

Psychiatric Council of the Joint Commission on Accreditation of Hospitals.''

It would seem to me that the author and reader will need to think of, if not explore, a number of factors before proceeding from this point: (1) to know the current and imminent socioeconomic-political picture, for this is the setting in which the choice is to be made; (2) to know the current "psychiatric scene" and its probable direction as they will affect the contemplated choice; (3) to know the socioeconomic-political picture and "psychiatric scene" in the formative years of the author, some thirty to thirty-five years ago, and contrast them with those of the young physician trying to launch his career today. This would seem to require a knowledge of the author's training background, his "generation" of psychiatrists, the reason he chose the field of psychiatry, his development, and how and why he finally got into the "career" of the proprietary psychiatric hospital "business"; (4) to know what the "young doctor of today" emphasizes and values in contrast, perhaps, to what the author does; (5) to recognize the "gap" between the author and the reader, that is, the current "gap" between the "teacher" and "student"; (6) to bridge that "gap," if possible, if only by recognizing and clarifying its existence; and (7) to recognize from the start that this can be no easy task, yet hope that the effort will be of some use to the reader faced with making his choice of a career.

Before launching into even a limited exposition of these factors, I would first like to express some of my own assumptions about physicians in general. I assume that, by and large, doctors are well motivated, that they choose "medicine" because they want to help "the sick," that at least as with "my generation" they have an "economic motive" too, and that this latter motive may not be as strong today among the "new breed" of doctors who have not known the lean years of the "great depression." Nevertheless, whatever the "motivation," it is so strong that the young medical student, and later doctor, has been willing to put the best years of his life into a crushing, competitive "grind" for at least five to ten years after gaining his bachelor's degree, to extend himself to the ultimate, to be tested and retested and thereby face failure at every turn, and further, to "invest" a great deal of money in the process, simultaneously surrendering the opportunity to earn during this long period. Aside from the emotional investment, we may roughly estimate the cost to be $100,000.

It would seem to me that a doctor must be very well motivated, but unwise, if he thinks that he will earn enough to compensate him for these years of emotional, physical, and financial sacrifice, let alone the emotional drain on him once he is launched on his "career." In recent times, of course, it is said that one often elects the field of medicine "to escape the draft." In all fairness, however, it seems more likely that many of the "new breed" of doctors enter the field with loftier motives in mind. I assume further that the medical student must derive some joy from his studies, and experience some anticipatory pleasure at the prospect of practicing his profession. He may also foresee the joy of spending the earnings of his busy practice, when it permits him the time to do so. If he is realistic, of course, he will be mindful of the relatively short life span of the "busy doctor."

I stress these assumptions to emphasize that the individual who successfully undertakes such a task will very likely excel against the described odds should he elect to work in the proprietary psychiatric hospital field. This would be especially true if he sees the following professional and personal, as well as monetary, advantages in it. As a resident-in-training he can gain excellent preparation for the office practice of psychiatry. There is a great difference in the total approach to the treatment of the self-paying patient and his family, as opposed to the publicly supported, or "teaching," patient. This may be unfortunate, but the reasons are obvious. There is the evident advantage of being able to individualize—to select one's patients—and to avoid the interference from government agencies to which the private nonprofit hospitals are increasingly subjected. There are opportunities for research and the freedom to try new approaches to therapy and administration. Some see an advantage in the very "challenge" which the proprietary hospital itself presents. Needless to say, the main advantage is an opportunity to set the best example in clinical psychiatry. It may be said that the proprietary psychiatric hospital has survived and succeeded against many odds because it has been able to maintain its autonomy. It has not had to face the constant dilemma of the private nonprofit hospital, namely, how to "survive on government subsidy and still remain autonomous."[2]

There is an old saying that "money talks." When the government supports building, research, teaching, and treatment programs in the university and voluntary hospitals, it speaks "loud and clear." It influences the autonomy and programs of these institutions in some obvious and numerous subtle ways. Accordingly, they are sometimes hardly as private (nonpublic) and autonomous as they may appear to be or like to feel. When the government suddenly suspends its support its "silence" speaks with a deafening and devastating effect. We are only too well aware of the crushing effect curtailment of funds has had on the training, treatment, and research programs of our medical school and voluntary hospital programs. It may be, then, that the proprietary hospital is just as well off to struggle to be self-supporting, so that it may remain more truly autonomous and stable in its program direction.

As already indicated, some authorities in recent years have begun to see the advantages for patients in proprietary psychiatric hospitals. California has been placing some of its state hospital patients in proprietary hospitals. This seems to have been of economic advantage. Texas has begun the same practice, and most recently the New York State Department of Mental Hygiene has begun a series of meetings with its proprietary hospitals. It is hoped that these meetings will lead to similar fruitful ends. Of great significance is Eli Ginsberg's recent recommendation to the state of New York that it "permit a corporation to practice medicine for profit."[3] He has joined an increasing number of people who believe that such practices "could provide good quality care at a price considerably below the average." This is another indication that responsible authorities are turning to the proprietary sector of psychiatric hospital practice because of its professional and administrative skill in providing quality care at reasonable costs. Most recently, the United States Congress has acted favorably on legislation containing a "mortgage-insurance program for investor-owned hospitals," which permits them to apply for mortgages. Though this has not become law, it certainly seems like a favorable straw in the wind.

At this point, I can return to the seven factors mentioned previously. I have little more to add about the socioeconomic-political settings, past or present, except to note that the author's "generation," in contrast to the younger reader's, is not quite the same. I am a psychiatrist who has observed the simple truth that the thinking, personality, and mental health of human beings are molded by their total experience. My psychoanalytic training and office practice were preceded by some years of state hospital experience in the early 1940's and capped by 20 years of experience, founding, and directing a highly specialized proprietary hospital program.[4] I have concluded that mental disturbance grows out of "sick" human experience, and may be reversed in a healthier social setting. A proprietary psychiatric hospital may furnish this new experience for a patient, in order to allow him healthy growth as well as symptom alleviation.

I believe that the above is particularly true in functional illnesses, and I strongly suspect that social factors play a role in shaping the symptomatology of organic illnesses as well. Because of my medical training, I keep an open mind about a possible physical basis for schizophrenia. It is possible that a real "breakthrough" will be made in this area some day, and then we will have the "cure." The fact that the modern "miracle" drugs alleviate symptoms should not be taken as positive proof that the basis of schizophrenia is physical. I think further that it would be wise to acknowledge the fact that any "cure" by physical means will not exclude the important role of the individual's social experience.

I am convinced that the discovery of the cause and cure of schizophrenia, our major and most prevalent mental illness, will not be found in my lifetime, nor in the lifetime of the current reader seeking his career. This is said despite the great emphasis on community psychiatry as our "salvation" and the "hope" that is held out because of our "modern drugs," both of which are making the current "psychiatric scene." I cannot be carried away by these because I have seen too many "cures" and "hopes" become mere palliatives which disappear, only to be succeeded by new "straws" that psychiatry grasps. On the basis of such experience, it would seem wise to be cautious, but realistic, and to avoid pessimism. A measure of optimism must be maintained if we are to have any success at all.

In the last 30 years or so, I have seen many "minor" and "major" discoveries hailed as the answer to our problem, only to see them fail, be discredited or abandoned, before they were fully tested, because of our impatient quest for "the answer"— sulphur-in-oil injections, insulin-coma and subcoma shock therapy, electroshock therapy, combined insulin-electroshock therapy, intravenous ether therapy, the tranquilizing and psychoactivating drugs, megavitamin therapy, and now "community psychiatry." I recall very well how insulin-coma therapy was hailed as the treatment which would almost make state hospitals unnecessary. Today, "community psychiatry" seems to be lowering the census of some state hospitals, and being used by those leading the assault on all psychiatric hospitals. However, this is no proof that these patients are being cured. It probably means that we have additional ambulatory sick people. This point is very well made by Klerman,[5] who says, "The history of mental health programs shows cycles of reform and decay, of promises made and expectations unfulfilled. Therapeutic claims have often been unsubstantiated by experience and experiment. Our current knowledge of the nature, causes, and treatment of mental illness, while significantly advanced over previous decades, is still inadequate to validate comprehensive programs of prevention and treatment. Given this situation research is continually required to test the validity of new ideas and to establish the efficacy of new treatments."

In the midst of the "psychiatric scene" of "my day" one must highlight the major role of psychoanalysis, and the passion with which it was promoted to project an understanding of psychodynamics and the causes and cure of psychopathology. The effect of this discipline, with its emphasis on instincts and intrapsychic forces, can hardly be measured in terms of the impact it had on psychiatric thinking, research, and practice.

This influence continues in the current psychiatric scene, though to a diminishing degree, as increasing emphasis is placed on social forces and extrapsychic factors.

The fate of the proprietary psychiatric hospital has been discussed and foretold many times. In most instances, dire consequences have been predicted for it, and even its relevance has been questioned. The idea that profit should be made from the care of the sick, particularly the mentally ill, seems to be associated with feelings of repugnance. I am sure that this often influences the judgment of the would-be prophets. However, as with everything else, he who would predict with any degree of accuracy must first have the power to foresee the future of our society and its value systems. Thus, it has been the purpose of this essay neither to predict the future of the proprietary psychiatric hospital nor to offer an opinion as to whether or not it warrants survival. My intention has been twofold—one, to render a general survey of the facts surrounding the proprietary psychiatric hospital toward the end of helping the reader make an intelligent choice about his career; and, two, to indicate and explore significant factors which I believe will determine whether the proprietary psychiatric hospital is "to be or not to be."

Gray's discussion of Kubie's paper,[2] "The Future of the Private Psychiatric Hospital," is of special interest and quite novel. She titles her discussion, "Does the Private Psychiatric Hospital Need a Future?" There is a certain appeal to her argument. She states that, "Since the voluntary hospital is tax-free and otherwise supported by tax-deductible endowments, and since it offers services only to the affluent or the interesting, it might best serve the general public by moving toward disbanding and disbursing its resources among the public hospitals." In an equally novel vein she suggests that these patients go to the proprietary hospitals which "desiring to remain outside of public control and admittedly profit-making, these institutions can attract patients by offering a type or quality of care very superior to that available anywhere else. . . . In response to this new demand many (of these proprietary hospitals) are continuing their growth to become advanced therapeutic organizations."

I have never heard this view expressed, and at first blush, I am not in agreement. However, should national health insurance compel voluntary psychiatric hospitals to accept all types of patients, and within limited catchment areas, on pain of losing public funds and their tax-free status, the recommendation of Dr. Gray could come to pass, but by government fiat rather than willing dissolution by the voluntary hospitals into the public system. Under any such conditions the effect on the viability of the proprietary psychiatric hospital is readily apparent.

Under national health insurance, however, there is bound to be a sacrifice of quality care for quantity care. This can be said safely without exercising a moral judgment and in the face of those who say that we do not suffer a shortage of doctors. They make unsupported claims of this nature, and indicate that the mere redistribution of our physicians would solve the crisis of insufficient services for the many. One can already hear with increasing stridency the charge that "American medicine" has provided best for the healers themselves—not for the sick—and that this situation must be rapidly reversed. Psychiatrists are most certainly not exempted from this charge. It is likely that better distribution would be salutary, though hardly a thorough solution, but how doctors would be redistributed in anything resembling a reasonable period is not yet suggested. However, a union leader recently declared, "It is about time that we placed the health of the nation ahead of the pecuniary interests of the health establishment."[6] As yet, too, it is not decided whether national health insurance will be managed by the government, with its bureaucratic faults, or the insurance companies, with their pecuniary interests. The resolution of these problems, of course, will have a direct bearing on the future of the proprietary psychiatric hospital.

Klerman,[5] in a further discussion of Kubie's paper,[2] attempts to promote "the community mental health era." Klerman makes the correct observation that most statistics are gathered from public institutions, thus indirectly criticizing the private hospitals for laxity in this area, although a recent extensive survey has emanated from a proprietary hospital.[7] He declares that, "it behooves all hospitals, whether public or private, to demonstrate that they are as successful as the home treatment or crisis intervention approaches." It would seem to me that it should be quite the other way around, particularly since these new techniques have hardly proven themselves as adequate, let alone superior, to hospital programs. Klerman states, "Although conclusive evidence is lacking, concern that regression and dependency are inevitable consequences of hospitalization is growing." This is digging up a dead horse long buried by the modern trends in hospital care. Klerman is right in asking "whether the private hospitals will restrict themselves to the direct treatment of those patients who can afford it, or involve themselves in the complex social processes subsumed under the umbrella of community mental health programming. The direction the private hospitals will take in this area will, of course, determine their future." The only fault I can find with Klerman's latter point is that he makes no reference at all to the proprietary psychiatric hospital—as though they did not exist—though they apparently admit more patients annually than do the voluntary private hospitals to which he addresses himself.

It is said that many, if not a majority of the young doctors of today, are quite different from those of a generation or even a decade ago. The present senior medical student may report that even the sophomore student of his school has a different outlook. At any rate, as a whole, the "young crop" of doctors seems to have entered medicine with a different outlook and different motives. They are doing their own thing, and seem to be more absorbed with the social-political scene. They are more receptive to national health insurance, group practice, and quality care for the masses. They do not seem to be as motivated by the economic as by the social aspects of the practice of medicine. They would seem readier than those of the "older generation" to be subsidized by the government, and then repay their debt by practicing in areas short of doctors. National health insurance will ultimately pay the tuition for medical school and draw on the qualified student of the poorer, rather than preponderantly from the middle and upper economic strata of society. In fact, very recently, a group of medical students in need of money at Wayne State University offered to indenture themselves to towns in need of doctors if these communities would pay their college expenses. According to the plan, the money would be repaid with interest and guaranteed medical service to the community for a stipulated period of time. Something of this nature was unheard of a generation ago. Naturally, if this is a fair assessment of the situation, the movement of doctors into the proprietary psychiatric hospital field will be affected.

How national health insurance is devised is certain to affect the proprietary psychiatric hospital. Should the federal government take full responsibility for supplying quality care to all of its citizens, and exclude the proprietary hospitals from its program, their lot will certainly not have been made easier. On the other hand, should it limit the hospital stay of a patient to a brief period there will remain a sizable demand for the hospital supplying quality long-term care. Proprietary hospitals exist even in England, where socialized medicine has held sway for a long time. Should our government make its plan very attractive to psychiatrists it could siphon off most of them, so that few would remain for the proprietary care of patients. In the past, however, public plans have not been very successful, and many believe that the anticipated "plan" in any form is not likely to do much better than current types of government-supported care.

However, another factor is present which needs to be taken into account: the people's awareness of its "right" to quality care, and its increasing courage to press strenuously for its due. It might influence the lawmakers to construct an unusually good plan which would "pool" most of the psychiatrists into the public hospitals. On the other hand, the public, if not the authorities, may press for care in private and proprietary hospitals of their own choice. At the moment, the public continues to learn, for instance, that most Blue Cross plans, private in nature, exclude it from care in any but psychiatric units of general hospitals. This, of course, gives the patient neither free choice of his doctor nor long-term care, even if it is indicated in preference to the short-term, or otherwise limited program of the psychiatric unit. Patently unfair, but true!

Of course, the ability of the current proprietary psychiatric hospital to maintain its standards and the fortitude of its medical people "to stick with it" will help determine whether or not the proprietary hospital will remain on the scene. Some psychiatrists have been "with it" for many years, and will either be retiring or see fit under the pressures to convert to a nonprofit status. On the other hand, if conditions permit, the corporations with their larger funds and business "know-how" may take over and even compete with the government for the skilled manpower needed to maintain quality psychiatric care.

When all is said and done, there is reason to suspect that the proprietary psychiatric hospital will survive, certainly as long as will any vestige of the free-enterprise system. Whether it will decline or increase in number is anybody's guess. The quality of its program will depend on the multitude of factors and vicissitudes mentioned and suggested above. In my opinion it would be sad to see them disappear from the scene. Quality psychiatric care could be the worse for it. In previous writings, I have suggested that the proprietary hospital be regarded and treated as a "public utility." It certainly serves the public and cares for our most precious commodity—the human being. As a public utility, it could remain "proprietary," be subject to controls and limitations of "profits" (as are the more usual utilities), and still have much-needed moral and financial support from the public—as long as it does a satisfactory job. Certainly if the government can see fit to subsidize airlines and loan monies to "save" bankrupt proprietary railroads and airplane manufacturers, it should not seem too radical an idea for it to assist public-serving proprietary hospitals, particularly since the need for bed space is dire.

On reflection, however, I am not so sure of this as I witness the deterioration of our "public" utilities. Further, I am now not at all certain that this would be a solution so much as an evasion of the problems of the proprietary psychiatric hospital. Perhaps they are the better off for them, derive their spirit and vitality because of them, and are thereby motivated to strive for superior programs.

REFERENCES

1. Group for the Advancement of Psychiatry. "Crisis in psychiatric hospitalization." 7:72 (March 1969).
2. Kubie, L. "The future of the private psychiatric hospital." *International Journal of Psychiatry,* 6:419 (December 1968).

3. Ginsberg, E. "Viewpoint: report of the Health Insurance Council." January 1971.

4. Gralnick, A., ed. *The psychiatric hospital as a therapeutic instrument: collected papers of High Point Hospital.* New York: Brunner-Mazel, 1969.

5. Klerman, G. *et al.* "Research aspects of community mental health centers." *American Journal of Psychiatry,* 127:7 (January 1971).

6. Taylor, W. J. *New York Times,* "Letters to the Editor," April 16, 1971.

7. Gralnick, A. *et al.* "Five-hundred case study in a private psychiatric hospital: further considerations in evaluation." *Psychiatric Quarterly,* 43:46 (January 1969).

Chapter 6
Development of the Clinical System

This chapter is the writer's attempt to summarize the development and essence of our thinking about the humanizing aspects of the psychiatric hospital. In doing so I have drawn on the ideas and writings of the authors, principally Frank D'Elia, and at times have actually paraphrased some of the papers contained in this book, as well as those in our first book, *The Psychiatric Hospital as a Therapeutic Instrument*. Admittedly, it is difficult to clearly trace and describe the evolution of some 20-odd years of experience, theorizing, and practice in a hospital.

High Point Hospital started with the theory that the psychotic patient was best treated by psychoanalytically oriented psychotherapy aimed at furnishing him curative "insight" into his intrapsychic problems. This would best be achieved in a healthier environment than that to which he had been accustomed. By force of circumstances the hospital soon found itself resorting for assistance to the physiologic and drug therapies. More importantly, it began to pioneer in the use of family therapy as an addition to strictly individual therapy; it has retained family therapy to this day as part of its armamentarium. However, it soon became incumbent upon us to clarify what we meant by a "healthier environment" and correct "hospital atmosphere." This led to our intensive study and refinement of the hospital's social structure into what we believed to be a valid therapeutic community. Thus we embarked on an exploration of the hospital environment and those extrapsychic factors affecting patients which finally led us to our present concepts and methods. It has been this continually changing quality of the hospital in its quest for better answers to the treatment of the mentally ill, particularly the schizophrenias, that has added to the difficulty in elucidating its evolution.

We wrote rather extensively for the literature, both on family therapy and the ingredients and use of the therapeutic community. The evolution of the latter concerns us most here. It was first channeled into new directions by combining the traditional occupational and recreational therapy departments in High Point Hospital into one group work department, with the emphasis on *group* and *working together*. Ultimately this was absorbed into the traditional nursing department which, with additional modifications, finally evolved into our social psychiatric nursing-therapy department. This consolidation promoted improved communication among all involved in patient-care and enhanced the community's therapeutic effect on the patient. Patients were increasingly committed to assuming responsibilities toward the hospital society in which they lived through the establishment of working groups with useful functions. This was the method. The concept was to expose their interpersonal problems to them and to us for study and solution. The aim was an environment whose elements were known and whose effect on the patient could be judged as positive, or healthy. The elements themselves could be described, understood, and duplicated. The total social structure could be seen as healthier and therefore therapeutic.

As our horizons expanded beyond the individual to include his family and the very hospital social structure in which he was immersed, with its own family of patients and personnel with whom the patient now lived, we logically moved from the idea of the *therapeutic community* to that of the *hospital as a therapeutic instrument*. The therapeutic community, as originally conceived, was an environment in which the patient could more easily become better or be helped by others to become well. The hospital as a therapeutic instrument was a society of individuals—both patients and others—so interrelated that the very social structure itself had a therapeutic impact on the patient. The two concepts were quite different and required dissimilar methods of implementation, let alone value systems. It had become our custom to speak of the *psychotherapeutic* rather than the *therapeutic* community; this, perhaps, was the earliest evidence of our ultimate destination, that the nature of the larger social relationships determined the individual's psychology. The family relationships were but mirrors of them, just as the hospital relationships were but reflections of those of the larger society in which the hospital existed. To the extent that the hospital personnel mirrored the better aspects and values of the greater society, to that extent did the patient have a better chance to improve, and vice versa. Furthermore, if we were to advance, our concentration would have to be on the larger social exchange systems rather than limiting ourselves to the dyadic and intrafamily relationships.

The concept of the humanizing influence of a hospital, in turn, seemed the logical evolution of this thinking, but for clinicians it was not as easy to come by. The concept was not as "scientific"; it seemed more consonant with such disciplines as sociology and philosophy. However, there has been much recently which forced one's attention on the concept. Society has increasingly been described as "sick" and "dehumanizing." Accordingly, the mentally ill were often thought of as dehumanized, and, sad to say, they often committed acts of violence which could only be characterized as less than human. Perhaps, then, the mentally ill had suffered some degree of dehumanization. Further, it was old and common talk that mental institutions, by their very nature, were dehumanizing. In the face of such constant attack on hospitals as being dehumanizing, there was good reason to explore and, if appropriate, question its justification.

The emphasis by psychiatry—and particularly by psychoanalysis—on the individual's intrapsychic structure and instincts as the root causes of the patient's illness was acceptable to the larger society and those responsible for its functioning. This is why "society" could tolerate and digest the extensive impact of Freud's theories despite their "distasteful" emphasis on sex and their threat to organized religion. As long as the individual was basically at fault, "society"—the larger exchange system—was absolved. The growth of family therapy, with its theory that the family was the "cradle" of mental illness, also permitted society to take this "therapy" to its bosom. Certainly, then, the family had to look to itself since it was the cause of the problem. Once more, society was absolved; it did not need to look into itself for solutions to individuals' problems—a belief which, it seems, is being demonstrated in contemporary politics.

Those who approach this subject tolerantly must accept, or agree with in some measure, the concept that the *community* rather than the *family* is the cradle of mental and emotional illness. They will further believe: that disturbed interpersonal relationships are evidence of social pathology; that "social relatedness"—that is, the way people as groups are related to each other—is important to their emotional and mental stability; that an alteration of social relationships in a healthy direction will reduce the production of mental illness; that the contradictory teachings of society lead to tensions severe enough to cause psychosis; that social conditions which are patently contradictory to the basic social beliefs and teachings under which we are acculturated cause personal conflict and emotional suffering sufficient to yield illness; and that conditions such as these take their toll on the "material" sufferers, as well as those who apparently are profiting from such situations. Those sympathetic to this viewpoint will believe that the polarization of people, no matter what the basis, is counterproductive and devastating to men's minds. They will see such conditions as tending to dehumanize the individual, that such dehumanization is related to the ·creation of mental illness.

If any of the above has even a bit of validity, then the psychiatric hospital has to take this into account in planning its "community," as such, to be therapeutic and in establishing its social relationships. Those in charge must believe that if the patient's environment contributed to his illness, then a "healthier" hospital environment will promote the restoration of more than merely a symptom-free state. On this basis our belief is that medicine and psychotherapy alone are powerless to do much more in the hospital than render the patient free of major symptoms. They are not likely to rehabilitate or radically alter his personality of and by themselves. If he has arrived in a somewhat dehumanized state, the hospital can only help him out of it by arranging its social relationships to restore the crushed human qualities and to generate the lacking ones, that is, to participate in counteracting the dehumanization process to which the patient had been exposed. This should be *the* function of at least some psychiatric hospitals, for there are some patients sorely in need of such service.

Thus there must be a broader view of the medical model of mental illness which takes the above into account and recognizes that medication, even when it is supplemented by psychotherapy, is limited without an environment which promotes personality growth and "humanization." In the many cases in which we in psychiatry have proved helpless, we have accounted for our inadequacy with such explanations as "the patient was too sick," "came to treatment too late," "he and the family did not cooperate," "he didn't stay in treatment long enough," and "the community rather than the hospital is the place for treatment." The last excuse is the current one, though sometimes we will admit to a degree of impotence as a profession. It may very well be that many of our failures are due to our limited view of the hospital's true potential and not the restricted resources of the institutions.

It was with ideas of this nature in mind that we began to evaluate our hospital environment in order to mold it into a valid therapeutic community. We agreed with Opler that the human personality was the end product of inherent potentials largely modified by its social experiences. Naturally one's human relationships were among these "social experiences," which could mold and remold his personality. However, this molding process was also determined by much broader and global sets of experiences not necessarily in the person's immediate environment, but which, nevertheless, might have a powerful impact on his personality. The problem was to determine which experiences developed the more "human" person. Was a happy home life all that mattered or could its effect be outweighed by the impact of gross injustice somewhere else when one had been raised to believe that "all men are created equal" and that none should suffer want in the presence of plenty?

Essentially we were in agreement that man's highest status as a human being was attained when he was unambivalently allied with others for the achievement of a worthy goal—not when he was isolated and working against such purposes. Certainly all of us in the hospital had a worthy goal (the health and humanization of the patient), but the problem was how to establish social experience and relatedness so that all could consistently agree on this goal, on exactly what it was, and so that all could work unequivocally toward its attainment. We believed that man's state was not inevitably the result of immutable forces, but one which was to a large extent subject to his determination and remedy. Accordingly, the state of a society's health—and, for that matter, the degree of humanization of its members—may be evaluated by the quality and magnitude of the elevating human values which tend to coordinate and integrate it. Opposed to these are the negative forces which strive to disorganize and divide it so that its members are ambivalent about these matters and thereby are estranged. Needless to say, then, the experiences to which the hospitalized patient is to be exposed are crucial. Our task is to determine what positive forces will prevail in the hospital and to remedy those which seem potentially to have a negative effect. Inevitably we will build a system of values into the hospital's fabric. The question is, who will determine it, and how, and how generally will people be brought to live by it?

The effective use of the hospital's social-group relationships is directed toward formulating and deciding on this value system and then promoting adherence to it. The total effort is intended to foster the patient's—and others'—ability to participate in the process and thereby advance his or their state of mental health. The "others" are the professional personnel who will likewise profit from the entire interchange.

In this respect the hospital may be regarded as a *psychotherapeutic community* because it can provide the patient with the same type of insight into himself and the kind of working through by guided experience that the dyadic therapeutic relationship may furnish. This is what likely happens with the healthy person in his everyday life experiences without his ever getting the insight furnished by a therapist. Perhaps his experiences have been healthier. At any rate, we are faced with thinking that the more positive and socially stable the hospital environment, the better the patient's chances are for a sturdier recovery. The nature of his experience with the group may promote personal growth, or it may destroy it.

The hospital may act therapeutically by constructing a series of social contexts, each more difficult than the preceding one, as part of its treatment plan. As he passes through each, the patient tests and strengthens his social skills. In this process he may acquire a realistic appraisal of himself, of others, and of himself in relation to others. Naturally his social adaptation will be better with such an acquisition.

In a manner of speaking, a psychiatric hospital should be the remedial society to which we turn to undo what the patient's environment has wrought upon him. As such it should be as devoid as possible of the injurious elements of outside society without being a refuge minus human problems and as filled with healing, humanizing resources as we can possibly conceive and implement. It is for us yet to discover whether there are common "human denominators" which account for our successes in hospitals which nevertheless differ a great deal technically. In truth, the "hospital" is a social system, a society with its own history, mores, and methods. The more highly these are coordinated, the more likely this society, as such, will serve a therapeutic, rather than an antitherapeutic, role. It is for us to discern one from the other, and naturally foster the first and discard the second.

As we defined and refined the ingredients of the therapeutic community and involved the patients as well as those who treated them in this process, we simultaneously implemented these ideas with changes in the social structure of the hospital. Essentially, the process was reciprocal; changes made in social relationships led to new ideas about what was necessary to the therapeutic community. In addition to our growing experience, the changes in the nature of incoming personnel—but more importantly, the changes in the nature of the patients, which was much more rapid—led to these new ideas and their implementation. It may be said that though changes in the value system also occurred, the basic core of it finally took on a certain stability which forestalled rapid fluctuations. It was noted that the involvement of the patients in this process had a therapeutic effect on them.

Several ingredients of the therapeutic community have already been suggested. Others are worth mentioning. A cardinal principle of such a hospital society is that its members *recognize reality;* thus the search for reality is constant. An outstanding symptom of the mentally ill, particularly the schizophrenias, is their impaired perception of reality. They are unaware that their perception is impaired, let alone the extent of it. A major task of the hospital, then, is to restore this sense of reality. It must be clear who determines and sets the boundaries of reality, and the nature of the social relationships established should also make this clear. In other words, the professional staff must be in a position of leadership which is flexible and the patient in an equally clear position as to who he is, and why, in relation to the therapeutic team. All relationships between these groups should constantly reflect this reality. No system of relationships which blurs this fact should be permitted. Though patients tend to be self-denigrating, affairs should be arranged so that their feelings of esteem flow from their living the role of patient; their status as being important comes from their ability to eventually recognize from the behavior of the staff that they are the sole concern of the devoted efforts of the staff. The staff, in turn, see their significance as arising from the quality of their performance in relation to the patients and their ability to assist the hospital community of which they are a part to fulfill its primary goal—the cure and development of the patient as a human being.

The very fine and constant control the professional team exercises over the hospital's social forces permits the paranoid patient to test reality against his distortion of it. He can do this without undue strain, which might destroy his defenses, but should he test unsuccessfully, the hospital structure is there to quickly correct the disequilibrium established by the failures. Thus the patient is enabled to try again and again until he is repeatedly successful. Naturally, the staff is there to foster and reinforce his every step in the direction of reality.

It is axiomatic that good communication is essential to the therapeutic quality of a psychiatric hospital. It must be well maintained not merely between the patient and his individual therapist, but between the patient and the patients as a group and the professional staff as a group—and the larger hospital community. Above all, this communication must be a continuing

process which leads to understanding and mutual trust, especially if it is to have a humanizing effect. Otherwise, it may be
nothing more than a mechanical exchange of words. How this
comes about between human beings is not exactly clear; how it
leads to their striving for the more, rather than the less, humane
in life is equally unclear. Doubtless, however, the achievement
of trust between the related parties is crucial, particularly since
paranoia and impaired judgment are so common among patients.
Naturally, these symptoms interfere with the attainment of good
communication and mutual trust. Another factor is the clinician's responsibility. For instance, if he is dealing with a suicidal
patient who wants a freedom or "privilege" which exempts him
from a surveillance the psychiatrist believes he still requires for
his safety, the clinician must deny it, although the patient may
interpret this as a lack of trust because he, the patient, has given
his assurance that he is no longer suicidal. At the same time, the
psychiatrist cannot trust this assurance. His clinical experience
tells him to be wary. Can trust ever be achieved under such
circumstances? Yes, of course; in the process of therapy and
interchanges between them, there will ultimately come improvement in the patient, trust in the doctor's integrity and judgment,
and trust that the patient is not testing and finally can be relied
on to fulfill his assurances.

If communication and its accompanying understanding and
trust are to reap rewards, respect and mutual goals must also be
reciprocated. These must develop not merely between the
patient and his therapist, but between the patient and his new
community, the hospital. Somehow there must be a harmony not
just in the dyadic relationship, but in the larger hospital relationships to which the individual is exposed, because their elements
also come to bear on him, sometimes quite heavily. So by the
same token, harmony within the family relationships will prove
inadequate to maintain emotional stability if there is gross
disharmony between the family's cohesive forces and the global,
external ones of a disruptive, contradictory, and tormenting
nature.

The patient enters the hospital with his own ideas about
whether he is ill, the nature of his disorder, how it should be
treated, and finally, when he is "well," to leave the treatment

relationship with the hospital. All of these ideas are likely to clash with those in whose hands he has been placed or has placed himself and on whom rests the responsibility for his health, if not his life, and that of others. Ordinarily it is the individual therapist, with his theoretical training and clinical experience, who brings his skills and powers of persuasion and manipulation, as well as his value system, to bear upon the patient. In office practice he does this alone, trying to bring the patient into harmony with his own ideas of health. When their mutual goal is reached, if not before, the patient is discharged as at least functionally cured.

In the hospital, which regards itself as and acts as a therapeutic instrument, the situation is quite different. The patient is not in the relatively simple dyadic relationship but a much more complex set of relationships. The difference is akin to the difference an individual experiences in his relationships to his small family as opposed to those he experiences in his relationships in the extended world. The skills and powers of persuasion of many are brought to bear on him. It is the value system of a *community* rather than an individual which affects him, and thereby more strongly. In addition, he lives in this community 24 hours a day for an extended period of time, constantly exposed to its effects. This is markedly different from the ambulatory office practice situation. It is also quite different for the hospital professionals who have continuing full-time responsibility for and exposure to the patient, rather than two or three hours per week.

To achieve our goals we must have long-term patients so that continuity and investment of the patient's time and energies in the environment are maintained. We must have a sufficient opportunity to act upon him therapeutically. Accordingly, a hospital such as ours cannot be a way station, a place where the patient just comes to "get well" or be "made well" in the traditional sense, but a place where he is going to live for awhile. He is not merely having a hospital stay during which some form of specific treatment will make him "well." The hospital is not a static environment in which he sojourns for a brief while or even "rests up and relaxes" for an extended period until he heals himself or heals with the aid of some specific agent. The patient does not come to this type of hospital merely to get rid of his symptoms, but to be basically affected in his orientation toward himself and others. The aim is not to make him as well as he once was, for that apparently was not well enough, but emotionally stronger than ever. The aim, of course, is to enable him to better withstand life's pressures.

In this type of hospital the patient's therapist is its agent, representing and attempting to bring the patient into harmony with its goals for him, its ways and aspirations for him, and its values, which are thought of as being healthy and health-producing life guides. Of course, there must be room for initiative, flexibility, and individuality for both the patient and his therapist, but it must be kept in mind that there are other professionals who are agents of the hospital community and attuned to its value system, standards of behavior, and methods of relating. They, too, bring their influence to bear on the patient. The constant, unavoidable struggle is to achieve as much common understanding of that goal for which we strive as is possible among those who influence the patient. This is the most difficult task. To the extent that it can be accomplished, however, to that extent is the hospital capable of functioning therapeutically as a total social group, or "instrument." In this regard, then, the patient also profits from this aspect of the personnel's interrelationships. The manner in which the patients as groups are interrelated will also influence the hospital's therapeutic quality. In essence, a general acceptance of an "approach" promotes a consistency which also adds a therapeutic dimension, provided that there is room for exploration of sound differences.

As has already been indicated, a hospital community, like any other social group, eventually acquires its own value system. The conscious use of this system to assist the patient examine his values, which may have contributed to his illness if not dehumanization, is another mark of a therapeutic hospital community. It is a measure of the hospital's therapeutic quality if it succeeds in helping the patient choose a value system, including the very one he may have and be ambivalent about, with which he may live in comfort, and which is somewhat consistent with that of those with whom he is currently related. If it is basically valid, as it should be in a "therapeutic" hospital, it should also serve the patient well later in his life. The danger to be avoided here is that the value system may deny the patient the ability to accept and participate in change. At any rate, he should have been engaged in a successful learning process of the hospital's social forces which showed him a possible need and gave him some choice in altering his values in a healthier direction. Thus his estrangement could give way to a healthy integration into the hospital society and later into the larger community, since the former is a reflection of the latter.

Recognition of the role of social factors in causing and curing psychopathology complicates the task of constructing a hospital system for the study and treatment of mental illness. The needed investment of human talent, resources, and energies is immeasurable and on a much greater scale than if the cause of such disorder is considered biochemical. It makes comprehensible the tendency of psychiatry to turn away from the perfection of our hospitals as social therapeutic communities. It is understandable, though deplorable, that we are compelled to pick the expedient rather than the promising, though more difficult, work of the "therapeutic" hospital. As a matter of fact, we seem to be increasingly turning away from hospital care itself to the community health center without any assurance that it will do better.

The therapeutic community is composed of individual systems and groups of systems which may be in relative harmony but which are more often in conflict. Never are they completely stable. The closer they approximate it, however, the better the therapeutic potential. The main responsibility for its achievement is that of the chief authority figure. His most difficult task is to be a strong authority figure without becoming authoritarian. He must combine the various systems and disciplines into a well-functioning unit, not merely create an atmosphere in which they may operate independently. His aim, especially with the professional disciplines, is for each to modify itself so that they may be welded into a therapeutic team. Each professional will have to sacrifice some part of his self-image, the aura of his own discipline, and the way he operates within it. He bases his self-esteem on them and thinks that without him, the patient would somehow not do well. This is what keeps professionals compartmentalized, rather than integrated, as a team. The chief authority, preferably medically and psychodynamically trained, should be experienced in working with other disciplines and thus be aware of and sympathetic to their ideas and goals. He should have a social orientation about the etiology of mental illness and its alleviation. At the same time he should be familiar with the physiologic and chemical treatments, appreciate their value, and be open to their use.

High Point Hospital probably went through these stages of development; its concepts and methods for their implementation changed, and we began to see the full extent of the patient's relationship to those other than his individual therapist. Their impact as larger social exchange systems could no longer be minimized to maintain the exclusive position of the dyadic relationship. Neither could the hospital's value system, as a potent force affecting the patient, be bypassed. The conclusion was inescapable that powerful human forces were at play in our social structure and that they affected the very human qualities of the patient, not merely his psychiatric symptoms. This became even clearer as we defined the ingredients of our community and finally saw them to be those critically important in the acculturation process which humanized the infant human being during his development. Naturally, such thoughts clarified further our changing view of patients and their treatment. Further clinical experience seemed to substantiate our concepts. For better or worse, the humanizing aspects of any hospital had to be explored. This might help explain why some patients mysteriously got well regardless of the type of hospital program, why some responded to one program rather than another, and why some seemed unresponsive to *any* program.

This subject is a proper area of consideration for the hospital psychiatrist, if for no other reason than that the dehumanizing aspects of hospitalization have been discussed with a passion and propaganda-like quality almost intended to produce public furor so that two things would follow: one, that the process of dehumanization would be seen as an inevitable component of psychiatric hospitalization and that such care would be without any redeeming features; and two, that it would be held unscientific, if not almost unreal, to question this concept. In considering this topic one must face some questions. What are the special factors present in a hospital which are supposed to contribute to the patient's dehumanization? Have they been scientifically and clinically proven to dehumanize the patient? Have they really been so prevalent, particularly in recent years, as to justify characterizing all hospitalization as being dehumanizing? Or has something of a myth been perpetuated for reasons that are no longer sound? Further, are we content with and certain of our understanding of what *dehumanized* really means? Are we aware of whose standards they are and satisfied with the measuring standards used?

The same, or similar, questions may be raised about the humanization of the hospitalized psychiatric patient. We are talking of a quality or dimension of the human being and must differentiate between the normal human being and the humanized or dehumanized individual. Returning the mentally ill person to a normal, or symptom-free, state is not necessarily synonymous with his humanization. By the same token, then, the patient who gets sicker in a hospital is not necessarily dehumanized by the hospital. These distinctions are not easily made.

In any event, all of this must be seen in the context of our current society and our hospitals in the main as microcosmic reflections of it. As already indicated, it is not uncommon for us to speak of our society as "sick" and of many of its citizens as "dehumanized." It is far from clear, however, that all who speak in this vein have similar definitions and concepts in mind—all of which adds to the complexity of the subject and increases our need to clarify the issues. Our burden is all the heavier because we are obliged to face the issues and yet remain within our area of expertise as clinicians in psychiatry. It would be much easier if we could wander off into areas other than our own, such as sociology, anthropology, and philosophy.

The psychiatrist may still assume that the study and treatment of the mentally ill is his concern, that logically, the determination and study of what is mentally "normal" is also his province. He may assume that his knowledge can contribute to the creation of "normal" human beings. However, the extent to which he will accept as his area of expertise the determination, study, and contribution of knowledge toward the creation of the "humanized" human being is questionable. This is understandable since, as yet, psychiatrists do not have even common under-standing about the origins and treatment of psychopathology; they disagree about the exact areas to which all should devote their treatment efforts.

We believe there is a clinical method of hospital treatment which helps the patient recognize the need to acquire certain humanizing qualities and which assists him in their pursuit and development. The technique includes the structuring and use of the hospital's staff as a therapeutic or human instrument in itself, in relation to the patient. It requires an ever-expanding knowl-edge and refinement of our therapeutic responses "as people" to the behavior of the mentally ill in the hospital setting. This is quite different from an improved understanding of the patient's intrapsychic forces and its conveyance to him. It involves the arousal of the patient's awareness of the pathology of his rela-tionships to others through the very nature of his relatedness to them in the hospital, both patients and staff. Simultaneously it involves exposure of the patient's values, both positive and negative, and how the latter injure his efforts at healing. This evolves from a comparison of his self-defeating values with the clinically selected constructive ones of the hospital community. Thus the "living relationship" to which he is deliberately exposed in this type of hospital contributes to his humanization. This is to say the person who ends up with the greater number and higher degree of positive values is the more "humanized" individual, and is healthier for it. Naturally, he will not arrive at such a state in three to four weeks of hospital care directed at merely relieving his florid psychiatric symptoms.

The hospital which aspires to affect patients in this manner and has the conviction that this is "therapeutic" develops con-cepts of what is "humanizing," in contrast to "normalizing." In addition, its techniques will acquaint the patient with the fact that the exercise of a humanizing influence on another is, in turn, humanizing and conducive to mental health. It is not merely a matter of how one is treated, but, equally important, how the patient treats with another. We recognize that this approach is part of our own value system. It has not sprung from thin air, but from our method and clinical experience with the hospitalized patient.

It is a truism that people think of one as being more *human* (humanized) if he enjoys positive relations with others, in contrast to the one who does not. The former has an abundance of certain qualities the other lacks. For instance, he is thoughtful and sensitive to others, kinder, altruistic, and so on, whereas the other is selfish, insensitive, and sadistic. There are numerous other qualities which help us contrast people. It is, of course, easier to do in extreme cases. We can easily think of the mass murderer as being less human, or "dehumanized," and unhesitantly think of him as being "sick." We use the words almost synonymously. In many cases, however, the synonymity is not readily apparent, though it is, nevertheless, there if we attune ourselves to see and accept it. This is similar to the difficulty we have in detecting the earliest symptoms of schizophrenia and accepting them as such. It is hard on the emotions to label someone with this diagnosis. It is no less so to mark a fellow human being as being less than human, or dehumanized. In the light of our growing clinical experience, however, it no longer seems necessary to defend the thesis that the more "human" person is the healthier and that it is within our province to treat the patient with this in mind.

This approach to patient treatment compels us to face several questions. What are the origins of the qualities which determine the degree of one's humanness? Are they genetic or social? Why do they vary so widely among people and sometimes so much within the same person? If environmentally determined, why are both positive and negative human qualities found in all levels of society and in varying degrees regardless of the social level? Why in this advanced society are the negative qualities on the increase and psychopathology so prevalent? Could there be a relationship between these facts? What effect is there on our psychology as we are exposed constantly to inconsistencies between what we see and do and the values on which we otherwise learn to rest our sanity? None of us has definite answers to these queries, but we can be quite sure that they are related to the mental status and humanness of people.

In another way, we may say that we are interested in the patient's human development. This requires close study of relationships and the manner of interreaction of both patients and staff, as individuals and as groups, and then interrelating them as social systems in ever-improving ways which evoke and develop the best in them. It is the essence of our hospital clinical technique and is accomplished with a focus on *human* qualities— what they are, who has them and who lacks them, how they may be acquired and developed. In turn, this can be done only in an organization of people devoted not simply to expunging symptoms, but more to an unabashed examination of the reality of their situation. The true role of each must be determined, known, accepted, and played to its fullest for the achievement of a sense of self-esteem. These elements comprise the hospital's social structure. In this living process, which is really "the hospital," symptoms will disappear and more human qualities will emerge. In this hospital setting, functioning effectively and functioning *humanly* are the same thing. This should not be equated with the humanitarian approach wherein "love and kindliness" are considered the great healers. The accepted objective is one's work well done by and for everybody, and this often requires quite different concepts and tools of treatment.

Our hospital has sought to add another dimension to the ordinary medical model. It is of a social order and in keeping with the concept of social psychiatry. However, it is not designed or directed to discard the medical model, but instead, to reinforce and update it in the area of psychiatric hospital treatment. We firmly believe that psychiatry is a medical discipline, just as other branches of medicine have remained, despite their having taken serious note of social and ecological factors which affect their area of expertise. Most of our patients need more than to be made symptom-free; they need to be humanized to repair society's damage, which has dehumanized them to some degree. This process of repair must take place in a psychiatric hospital with an added social dimension—one which uses its professionals as a therapeutic instrument and a humanizing force.

PART TWO
CLINICAL APPLICATIONS

Chapter 7
The Problem of Primary Change in Psychotherapy and Psychoanalysis: Repair versus Reconstruction

by Maurice H. Greenhill, M.D.
and Alexander Gralnick, M.D.

In the course of psychotherapy, the therapist is dealing concurrently with several parameters of intrapsychic forces, interactions, and technics involving both the patient and himself. His goals, or end points, are variable and flexible, although grounded upon predictions, always taking into account what is possible for the patient. Sooner or later he is compelled by the reality of time, nature of the psychopathology, rational demands of the patient, or an acknowledgment of his own limitations or the limitations of the science to delineate his ultimate goal with the patient. As a therapist with a given patient, what has he sought or what has he wrought?

Freud's statement that "The business of analysis is to secure the best possible psychological conditions for the functioning of the ego; when this has been done, analysis has accomplished its 'task,'" sets a general ground rule for the final objective. But "the best possible . . . conditions" fall upon a broad spectrum of achievements ranging through amelioration, palliation, repair, and reconstruction. We have come to believe that the results of psychotherapy are weighted toward the pole of the spectrum denoting amelioration, while those of psychoanalysis are at the opposite pole characterized as reconstruction, although in either instance results may settle anywhere on the range depending upon particular circumstances. In any event, to accomplish or restore the functioning of the ego denotes *change,* change in symptoms, away from symptoms, in interpersonal relations, attitudes, thought processes, values, in the balance of intra-psychic forces, or in any other dimension of behavior necessary to achieve this goal. Dysfunction is corrected, decompensation modified to equilibrium, or basic traits reconstructed in quantity or quality.

What then are the ultimate goals the therapist sets or settles for with his patient? Are they in the area of reparation (amelioration, palliation, correction of dysfunction, restoring equilibrium in the function of the ego) or reconstruction (modifying or reforming basic traits)? And in the transactions of psychotherapy what precisely produces *change* in the direction of health? It is essentially these questions to which we address this presentation.

We have already indicated that one ultimate goal is reparative or restorative, to permit the patient to function as he once was or to provide realignment of existing traits in order to produce more useful, less destructive, reactions to stress. This can be called *secondary change.* Change is implicit in this area, but it involves less sweeping movement and modification in id forces, defenses, ego structure, and conflicts. Some degree of reconstruction occurs here *sui generis,* but the result is largely *reparative.* In general, secondary change connotes "repair" or the amelioration of conflictual anxiety toward restoration of function.

It may be said that all psychotherapeutic endeavors have as a common goal the accomplishment of secondary change. Whether it be advice, persuasion, "support," manipulation of the environment, or dealing with unconscious motivation and transference phenomenon, the amelioration of conflictual anxiety may result. This is not accomplished by any one factor, such as "insight," "corrective emotional experience," "emotional support," or the resolution of a "transference neurosis." These, as well as other factors, are at work individually, severally, and with varied timing. The process is complex and includes combinations of identifiable methods and interaction phenomena such as uncovering of defenses, ventilation of feeling, dealing with conflictual anxiety, assimilation of therapist's attitudes, desensitization of transference struggles, working through resistances, and interpretation. Such methods are designed to produce an effect upon the patient which, in order to identify a therapeutic formula, has been called "insight," "corrective emotional experience," or "resolution of neurotic conflict." There is much evidence in the literature and in the experience of psychoanalysis that these factors represent concepts of dynamic interaction which produce change.

And what is the end point of such change? We as therapist or the patient select the end point, deciding for the present that a practical goal has been reached. Most often, secondary change has been achieved, some stage of amelioration which allows the ego to function for the present. At the same time the patient may give indications that he may deal with pertinent stresses in the future with less neurotic or more appropriate responses.

Freud has stated that the end points in analysis are determined by effect of traumas, constitutional strength of the instincts, and modification of the ego (altering of defenses). Ferenczi indicates that ultimate goals have been reached when "In every male patient the sign that his castration anxiety has been mastered must be forthcoming, and this sign is a sense of equality of rights with the analyst; and every female patient, if her cure is to rank as complete and permanent, must have finally conquered her masculinity complex and become able to submit without bitterness to thinking in terms of her feminine role." Freud comes to the same conclusion: "We often feel that, when we have reached the wish for a penis and the masculine protest, we have penetrated all the psychological strata and reached 'bedrock' and that our task is completed. And this is probably correct."

But it is common experience that not infrequently all the stated end points are reached and sufficient amelioration has not taken place to justify appropriate functioning of the ego. Secondary changes have transpired, but therapy cannot stop or must be reinstituted because illness continues to intervene. We are here compelled to cope with a movement into primary change.

We are not implying that primary change means a wholesale

reconstruction of character traits. We are suggesting that as a result of dealing with another end point, the tenacity of nuclear conflict, a basic reorientation in all psychological strata takes place which permits a result closer to a "cure" for certain patients.

Before discussing nuclear conflict we wish to go on record that we cannot with satisfaction accept the concept of reaching bedrock at the levels Freud postulates. Analysis can proceed no further, according to him, if the constitutional strength of the instincts is excessively strong. He states: "The quantitative factor of instinctual strength in the past opposed the efforts of the patient's ego to defend itself, and now that analysis has been called in to help, that same factor sets a limit to the efficacy of this new attempt. If the instincts are sufficiently strong the ego fails in its task." In another context he writes: "We can well believe what our daily experience suggests that the outcome of an analysis depends principally upon the strength and depths of the roots of the resistances constituting the ego modification. Once more we realize the importance of the quantitative factor and once more we are reminded that analysis has only certain limited quantities of energy which it can employ to match against the hostile forces."

Freud also claims that the strength of hereditary defenses is an additional factor which constitutes an end point. These defenses include "adhesiveness of libido," "mobility of libido," "loss of plasticity (exhaustion of capacity for change and development)," and "strength of primal instincts (death instinct and Eros)."

There is little doubt that all of Freud's factors must be taken into account. Nevertheless it is common experience in our time that we as therapists are confronted with problems of chronicity in psychopathology which demand additional exploration beyond these end points.

THE POSTULATE OF NUCLEAR CONFLICT

We are impressed by the fact that at "the end point" and at "bedrock" the patient confronts us with a constellation of mechanisms to which he clings desperately and beyond which he cannot seem to go. This constellation might be called "nuclear conflict" and is largely unitary and specific for the patient. It represents the basic primitive solution for infantile conflict, hardened and habituated by conditioning throughout most of life. It is the "master cell" commanding the action of the defenses and is at the matrix of character structure. In one instance it is tenacious symbiosis, in another pure oedipal conflict coloring all life situations, and in another "castration anxiety." In prolonged therapy in chronic states the patient himself comes face to face with his nuclear conflict in naked form. He recognizes it, verbalizes it, associates on it, evinces deep feeling over it, but despite all of this continues to operate with it. With all of his awareness, he undergoes certain clinical manifestations which will be discussed later.

This, in effect, is the end point previously described in the literature. Now both the challenge and the reality compel us to go beyond this.

CLINICAL ASPECTS

This problem was brought to our attention through the question of "interminable analysis." In dealing with chronic cases, both in the private practice of psychiatry and in private hospital psychiatry, we have been afforded the opportunity of "staying with" chronically ill patients because there has been no other choice, i.e. the patients were in such discomfort that they consistently had to be under treatment. The ambulatory case load of one of us (MHG) consists largely of patients "after-analysis," namely, those who had been discharged from psychoanalytic treatment. Some had returned for further work with the same analyst, but chose eventually not to return after further exacerbations. Others, because of circumstances or negative transference, had not gone back to the initial analyst. Still others had had three or four analysts previously.

We have concentrated on 15 such patients in order to formulate our method. Each one of these had "completed" analysis with a reputable analyst who was at least a member of an official analytic association or prominent institute. All patients have been in therapy at least six years and two for 20 years consistently. The average length of time in therapy has been 9.8 years. These are all experienced sophisticated analysands who function in life and handle most crises well, but who are frequently plagued by reactions to special crises. These were found to be intimately related to their nuclear conflicts.

Another group of patients considered methodologically were 15 individuals who had been hospitalized at the High Point Hospital for chronic schizophrenia or borderline states. These had had therapy or analysis of three years' duration or longer. A striking clinical feature was the immediate exposure of the nuclear conflict in which the patient continuously attempted to keep the conflict in his hands rather than in the therapist's through the use of last-ditch defenses such as symptom defenses and communication devices. The patient had taken control to such an extent that institutionalization had taken place for up to two years during which each had at least three hours of therapy per week.

THE METHODOLOGY OF HANDLING CHRONIC STATES

We then came to the consideration of the nuclear conflict as the gyroscope of chronicity. There is an obsessive quality, a repetitiveness, a hard core of fixation on a "last-ditch" pattern that is the *leitmotiv* of the patient's psychological function. This is the principal determinant of character traits. By a continuous conditioning process, symptom reactions serving to preserve this nuclear pattern become fixed in chronic form.

How does one approach this chronic state in an attempt to reconstruct it? The patient has reached an "end point" at which he stands face to face with his nuclear conflict. What is striking is the degree of insight which he has achieved at this point. This is emotional insight. He verbalizes it with strong feeling; there is an aura of desperation in his productions, with expletives of frustration, with despair, tears, often deep depression. He arrives at the place where he always describes himself as two persons, the one the skilled analysand aware of his ego functions and defenses, the other an infantile primitive being dissociated from his ego. He abhors the latter as he gets to know it but is imprisoned by it. He is clearly in a dissociated state, in which part of him watches anaclitic experience in the other part of him without at first being able to exercise control over it.

REITERATION IN FOCUSING ON NUCLEAR ANXIETY

One goal of the therapist is to bring the dissociated state into clearer focus. In doing so he must be prepared to tolerate the anaclitic, or primitive, reactions of the patient, because these are often more painful to the therapist viewing them than to the patient. In doing so the therapist brings the patient back again and again to the material of the nuclear conflict. He compels the patient to reiterate the details. When the frustration of the patient in not being able to achieve movement in the conflict becomes unbearable, the therapist lets up for one session or two, but invariably returns to it. He chips away at this hard core in this fashion, approaching it again and again, from one vantage point or another. The activity of the therapist is not as great as it sounds; he is not overwhelming the patient. By this time resistance to communication is no longer encountered, only resistance to change. The therapist simply has the patient stay on the topic.

We acknowledge that there is a measure of awkwardness in this method. The truth is that we as psychotherapists have not yet learned how to treat the patient in this area of chronicity. What is required is an investigative approach to test out pushing beyond set frontiers. We seem to be bound by our traditional belief that awareness or insight is the cure. In these cases profound insight of an emotional nature, not an intellectual one, appears obvious, yet the patient remains imprisoned in the grip of his fundamental conflict. An entire dimension remains unexplored, whatever it is. It may have something to do with conditioning or learning or with the absence of any other type of experience in the patient's life. He knows of no other way to react. Perhaps at this point in the therapy we must attempt to free ourselves of the concept of the unconscious or to stress it less and bring to bear additional theoretical models related to conditioning or learning theory or cultural influences and values or something as yet undiscovered without complete capitulation to traditional forms of unconscious motivation.

SETTING LIMITED GOALS FOR NEW MATERIAL

The process of confronting the nuclear conflict is a slow one. The patient clings tenaciously to his basic complex and yields slowly after months or years. It is especially important to the therapist in his inevitable frustration in dealing with this bedrock chronicity to know that he has a logical technique at hand in which time is relative. *The basic technic with any chronic process is focusing upon the fundamental problem plus setting limited step by step goals toward an ultimate objective.* We hold that this is true throughout medicine.

One cannot, of course, expect striking new material with any degree of frequency after years of analysis. In chipping away at the nuclear conflict one remains alert for clues, however sparse, which are related to it, with the goal of loosening it little by little. One has to be satisfied with limited goals, for what might have seemed trivial or redundant earlier in analysis may be a milestone in producing movement in chronicity. The clue may be a slight shift in emphasis, a diminutive lessening of emotional response, a genuine acknowledgment of a value previously resisted, a shift in character of associations, or slight modification in dream content. This last factor, dream content, has been found by us to be a most significant type of new material and frequently serves as a barometer in the slow process. In confronting the nuclear conflict we are meeting a stubborn last-ditch resistance which appears to be different from the resistances encountered earlier, namely those related to the ordinary ego defenses and transference. It appears to be an almost impenetrable armor working against fixed conditioning while the patient somehow believes there may be nothing to support him whatsoever should he yield.

A case in point is that of a woman who came to analysis at the age of 32 with depressiveness, a labile irritable character, obesity, and essential hypertension. Seven years later she was still working through her nuclear conflict, which was a tight symbiosis with her mother who had been dead 15 years. When analysis itself had become chronic, she lay on the couch during her sessions, making sucking noises and crying uncontrollably whenever her mother appeared in her associations. Whenever she sensed she might be relinquishing the symbiosis, she went on eating binges, reverting to types of food her mother had used as rewards to her in childhood such as noodles, frankfurters, and chicken skin. The types of leads to change and new material which seemed to be meaningful were limited to the context of the nuclear pattern, i.e. material on the sucking sounds, diminution of crying with mother material, changes in character of food ingested, and in particular modification in character of dream content. For example, the monotonous appearance of mother and food in dreams gave way to consistent appearance of women friends alternating with mother. Then the limited goal became the watchful waiting for other than mother material. Some time in the seventh year murderous men began to appear and the limited goal became the clarification of these. Eventually the patient became aware that these dangerous men stood for the therapist who was trying to "murder" her infantile anaclitic self.

Connected with the use of limited goals for new material is the role of interpretation. By this time patients spontaneously and freely offer interpretations and in this way collaborate in the loosening of the nuclear conflict. This is therefore encouraged, while at the same time the therapist becomes active in sharpening the interpretation to directly unearth the limited goal.

COMPELLING ACCEPTANCE OF THERAPIST'S VALUES

The patient brings to analysis psychological and cultural values which have contributed to the failure of ego function. These are fixed beliefs, attitudes, and actions which are used as guidelines for interpersonal relations. These are extremely resistant to change, as they are all the patient knows. They have been welded into the character by continuous stimulus-response experience and by unyielding pressure from the cultural group from which the patient comes. On the other hand, it is expected that the analyst has healthier values, both from his background and his professional training. Whatever his values are, it does not matter as long as they are healthier. Here is a parameter which can be used therapeutically. It is recommended that during the period of analysis leading to confrontation, the therapist identify the patient values, both healthy and unhealthy, as well as his own in juxtaposition to these, and be prepared to deal with them openly when he finally engages the nuclear conflict.

This, too, has to be done by repetition and reiteration. The particular nature of the therapeutic relationship and setting causes the patient to be vulnerable to change in values if only the therapist will consciously take advantage of this. Even the direct confrontation of nuclear forces by repetition is a new value which has been added.

In the hospital setting a particular opportunity to change values occurs. The studied values of the social structure of the hospital are forces differing markedly from the unhealthy values the patient brings with him from outside, and during the course of institutionalization his very presence among these values compels him to begin to live by them, if he is there long enough. When viewed in this way, our group of hospitalized patients profited in considerable measure from longer than shorter hospitalization owing to longer exposure to repetitive technique.

UTILIZING HEALTHY FACTORS

One occasionally hears the admonition "work with the assets of the patient." We have never been quite sure how this was to be done and for what purpose except for simple encouragement to relieve unbearable tension in the patient during critical periods in psychotherapy. Unless it was applied selectively in this way it seemed to have little meaning to us. While adhering to the production of movement in the chronic process, however, we began to be aware of the value of utilizing the healthy factors in the patient to surmount the infantile ones.

We should call attention to the fact, as so many others have done, that we as psychiatrists have been almost completely concerned with the negative factors in the patient's psychological function. The arduous task of unraveling and understanding pathology has largely dictated this. Perhaps more than any others, the psychobiologists under Adolf Meyer have called attention to the importance of identifying assets, but this was more for determining prognosis than for using it to technical advantage in their treatment plans, which they called "resynthesis." Psychoanalysis has been largely concerned with the genesis of symptom formation and its relationship to unconscious motivation, which necessarily gave priority to negative factors.

But in dealing with the hard core of the nuclear conflict, concern with the negative factors alone does not work. The patient can be brought to the most primitive level by focusing on the negatives, but when that is accomplished he cannot be constructively moved out of the anaclitic state by the negative approach alone. Such movement takes place by dealing with positive variables in the ego function rather than with negative ones, or with a combination of both.

To be specific, the utilization of healthy factors occurs at two points in the therapy of the nuclear conflict. The first takes place in phases of disassociation, i.e. when the patient himself is aware of two selves, the one attained as a result of therapy in which he functions appropriately, the other that part of him which he recognizes as infantile and nuclear but which he cannot relinquish. At those moments he feels helpless, frustrated, and desperate, and avows that there is no way of life to replace what he feels he must give up. At these points he must be made to feel the therapist's genuine acknowledgment and appreciation of his assets, which in the long run are the only factors that can fill the void left by resolving the nuclear conflict. The therapist does this by emphasizing healthy factors when the desperation is keenest or by refocusing on positive variables at these times.

The second point of utilization of healthy factors takes place whenever the exposure of nuclear conflict becomes critical in any context, at which time the therapist deals with positive and negative factors concurrently. Many of these patients with chronic disturbances have been accustomed to "double-bind" operations at the hands of key figures. In these instances the "double-bind" effected has been weighted on the negative side with a positive approach being subsidiary. We as therapists use this familiar mechanism, except that we emphasize the healthy factors while dealing with the negative. For example, we may deal with positive variables and the hostility of the patient concurrently by pointing up the fact that many demonstrate ambivalent feelings toward him and in doing so show strong positive feelings toward him while reacting to his hostility. In the hospital situation we demonstrate this fact by action in giving him group responsibilities while at the same time we explore in therapy his hostile primitive impulses in the nuclear conflict.

In many instances we do not know why dealing with healthy factors works, but we have observed that it does. We entertain the consideration that we do not have to be defensive about this, but rather that we must apply the spirit of inquiry to it.

THE SPECIAL NATURE OF THE PATIENT-THERAPIST RELATIONSHIP

In attempting to move beyond the end points prescribed for psychoanalysis, a fresh look at the physician-patient relationship has to be taken. Important and realistic as transference phenomena are, they are not sacrosanct and are subject to review. We hold that the therapist has to be prepared to deal differently with a relationship when "bedrock" has been reached and when he is endeavoring to produce primary change by subjecting the last bastion of psychopathology, the nuclear conflict, to erosion. Ever mindful of the implications of transference, in these situations he must extend the dimensions of the traditional concept of transference or, as it were, move *beyond transference*. This is a subtle point which could easily be misunderstood. Perhaps we might call it "more than transference" or "a different type of transference." Whatever we call it, it is a basic ingredient in chronic care.

The cornerstones of the relationship in primary change are the physician acting on the transference, special involvement of the physician, and the character of reliance on the physician. All of these features denote greater activity on the part of the therapist than is traditional. But this is very selective activity, largely nonverbal, and is expressed through an attitude of limited involvement brought to bear only when the nuclear conflict is yielding to resolution or whenever crises occur during this late stage of therapy. Such action attempts to convey to the patient that "we are concerned." It goes beyond the traditional detachment practiced when the therapist is interested only in the patient achieving insight.

When the physician acts on the transference, he is called on to maintain all elements in transference relationship technics, except that he permits some degree of his positive feelings for the patient to come through, selectively, in the "here and now" of crises in the therapeutic process. It is here that he deliberately acts as a parent in his own right regardless of transference distortions by the patient. In fact at these times it is as if he deliberately stands up to these distortions with his own strengths as an additional way of loosening the hard core of nuclear conflict. It is here that we go beyond the doctor-patient relationship as a ubiquitous method and look to ourselves. And here we must expose more fully to ourselves how we act with our positive feelings, our concerns for the patient, our firmness of limit-setting, and the impact of our value systems on his.

This implies involvement with limitations, but we do not shrink from this. It is involvement with the patient reality-based with positive overtones. Again the attitude of concern takes place only in specific situations of crisis as they occur in the "here and now." We allow that we too have an emotional investment in the therapeutic endeavor and that we intend to protect the patient when it is professionally indicated. We do not believe that this is the same as countertransference, i.e. we are not reacting to the patient with our own negative factors. What we are doing with limited involvement is not construed as being unhealthy; rather we consider such behavior appropriate to the professional role. If one thinks carefully about this, he sees that this technic is a basic one in treating chronic situations, whether it be schizophrenia, brain damage, or a chronic medical disorder. It reaches its greatest refinement in effecting primary change by working through nuclear conflict at the extension of end points for analysis.

Of course it may be said that this leads to greater reliance of the patient on the therapist, but what is wrong with that? We have long operated on the assumption that the patient must not be left with a transference neurosis, that he must be free, that he must be helped to achieve a state of absolute independence. This is not realistic. No patient is absolutely free after analysis. We are really referring to an ideal through which we hope the patient will resolve crises or follow guidelines from what we have incorporated in him rather than by physically turning to us. We cannot avoid the fact that we have implanted something of an image-ideal within him on which he is forever reliant to some degree. We count upon a type of reasonable appropriate dependency of this nature and seek to use it in dealing with nuclear conflict and in practicing this form of continuous care.

CONCLUSIONS AND RESULTS

We have presented the problem of primary change in psychotherapy and psychoanalysis through comparison of repair and reconstruction. With the ultimate goals of therapy placed on a continuum between repair and reconstruction, results are most often weighted toward repair which might be designated as secondary change. Whether or not primary change in intrapsychic forces takes place is problematical, and the extent of such reconstruction was questioned by Freud and others in terms of end points for analysis beyond which primitive forces within the patient would not allow the therapist to go.

In our time we are compelled by circumstances not to give up at this point. Increases in the incidence of character disorders, schizophrenia, and chronic medical disabilities, the development of community clinics and mental health centers, the knowledge that approximately 50 percent of psychiatric patients are seen in hospitals or clinics rather than in private practice, and social case work, welfare and antipoverty programs dictate that we must learn to cope with the problem of chronicity. We are not afforded the luxury of giving up on patients when we believe that we can do no more for them. We must find not only methods of continuous care but new ways to go beyond heretofore established end points in psychotherapy.

We have endeavored to explore one way of "pushing through" by evolving methods of resolving nuclear conflict. This is a bedrock constellation of forces which is left after defenses, resistances, and transference phenomena have been worked through. Insight has genuinely been established, yet the patient and therapist are left confronted by such nuclear forces as symbiosis, oedipal conflict, and castration anxiety.

Our method consists of a focused campaign against this hard core. This is accomplished by reiteration of such focusing, setting limited goals for new material, compelling the patient to accept the values of the therapist, utilizing healthy factors, and developing the therapeutic relationship beyond transference. Many of these factors have been intuitively utilized by professional personnel in dealing with chronic patients in all manner of settings, but we wish to call attention to these in a studied fashion.

In the process of attempting to effect primary change the patient is brought face to face with his nuclear conflict and views side by side his ego matured by years of therapy and his primitive anaclitic nature. This is a confrontation which is courageously faced by the therapist who utilizes his healthy values and concern for the patient to buffer the blows until a type of desensitization occurs.

Our subjects were 15 patients "after-analysis" in their seventh to twentieth year of analysis and 15 hospitalized patients with at least five years of therapy and two years of hospitalization behind them. The results are encouraging in that most of these patients have learned how to react to their own primitive complexes with reduced emotion and noticeable character modification. Such primary change is displayed in the ascendancy of positive traits and the surrender of tenacity and stubborn adherence to negative characteristics. None of the patients gave way to psychotic episodes while this aspect of treatment was practiced. None have given up their attempts to further improve. Some have continued to cling to their nuclear conflict, but all have changed to some degree in other respects.

It may be said that this is not a practical method because of the time involved, but there appears as yet no alternative to meeting the therapeutic demands of chronic patients other than to stay with the helping process. We also view this in the larger scheme of things as an investigative procedure which may lead to more practical measures in coping with chronic pathology and further technics of psychotherapy.

REFERENCES

1. Ferenczi, S. "Das problem der beendigung der analysen." *Int. Z. Psycho-anal.*, 14:1 (1928).

2. Freud, S. *Analysis terminable and interminable. Collected Papers*, vol. 5. New York: Basic Books, 1959.

Chapter 8
Recent Considerations in the Broad-Spectrum Treatment of Inpatient Schizophrenia

in collaboration with the senior author, Frank G. D'Elia, M.D.

Schizophrenia is a disease entity which is both baffling in nature and uncommonly complex. Although our hospital has devoted many years to the treatment of schizophrenia, we discuss this subject with a degree of trepidation. Sophisticated as we sometimes permit ourselves to feel, we nevertheless remain convinced that there is much more to be learned about schizophrenia than we now know.

We start with the assumption that schizophrenia is a functional mental illness which has its roots in pathologic relationships experienced at one time or another in life, probably early, but not necessarily so. While we do not exclude the possibility that schizophrenia may have its origins in some physiologic disturbance, our clinical experience teaches us that a pathologic environment sets off this self-perpetuating process which, once started, is most difficult to arrest, let alone reverse. We believe further that only a properly designed environment may arrest and reverse the process of schizophrenia. The correct social structure, then, will not merely expose the underlying forces of illness, but will permit existing healthier parts of the personality to gain ascendance and cause the emergence, if not a fresh beginning, of healthy qualities. Once in motion, these forces will lead to healthy behavior and normal judgment about reality; no longer will any abnormal intrapsychic forces be able to generate secondary symptoms, faulty judgments, and distortions of reality.

It is difficult to say something rewarding about the subject of schizophrenia in a relatively short space. Certainly the phrase "broad spectrum" suggests that many avenues of attack on the disease are open to us. And so they are! Let us enumerate some. Apart from psychotherapy, there is analysis, analytically oriented psychotherapy, and intensive therapy in both; milieu therapy, total push therapy, art therapy, recreational therapy, occupational therapy, music therapy, and work therapy; among the shock therapies are electroshock, insulin coma, and subcoma therapy; metrazol therapy, combined insulin coma and electroshock, carbon dioxide therapy, and a host of other similar therapies. Then, of course, there are the drug therapies, from the bromides to the tranquilizers to the psychic energizers to the mind expanders, and others involved in the sleep therapies. And not to be forgotten are family therapy in its various forms, from simple to concurrent to conjoint. Then, of course, there is outpatient therapy as contrasted with inpatient therapy, and individual therapy as contrasted with group therapy, not to mention individual therapy combined with group therapy—and omitting completely the question of whether the chair or couch is used in these. Finally we come down the list to pentothal therapy and hypnotherapy. This enumeration is not exhaustive; one can think of others, ranging from psychodrama to psychosurgery.

The word "treatment" which occurs in the title gives us some cause for hope. Though it is true that psychoanalysts generally believe that schizophrenia is not amenable to their highly refined skills, some at least would consider this disease subject to treatment. The fact, however, that there are so many treatments is cause for alarm. Our tedious enumeration of the many treatments available might seem amusing if we did not know that when we have so many types of treatment for one disease, we are dealing with a very refractory syndrome.

What of the phrase "inpatient schizophrenia"? Is there a suggestion that "inpatient" schizophrenia as an entity differs somehow from "outpatient" schizophrenia? Probably not.

However, the current emphasis on community psychiatry, let alone the universal reluctance to hospitalize the mentally ill until all other measures have failed, generally results in an "inpatient schizophrenic." This is true of the typical acute emergency admission. Much time has elapsed, and the acute situation is usually an exacerbation superimposed on a process already chronic. The disease has long been permitted to do its devilish work insidiously, and those who undertake its treatment within the hospital will have their task cut out for them. In this respect we may indeed have an "inpatient schizophrenia."

Over the years we have increasingly accepted and treated large numbers of "borderline" and schizophrenic patients. Today we tend to think in terms of "borderland" schizophrenia, the broad area of mental illness which tends to defy diagnosis as well as comprehension. Pathologic social interaction characterizes "borderland" schizophrenia. In our opinion, patients suffering such pathology are as psychotic as any with the usual frank stigmata of psychosis. We are just not yet accustomed to think in these terms, though they are as refractory to treatment as the obviously deluded and hallucinated.

In our earlier years of hospital practice the spirit of psychoanalysis thoroughly permeated our psychotherapeutic efforts. Understanding of our patients, always just within our grasp, continued to elude us. Psychologic tests recorded the existence of an oedipal complex, or of castration anxiety, and almost always the presence of a nuclear conflict. Some of our staff were trained analysts; others were in training or about to begin. We were following the courses and leads plotted by others. The patients should have been improving. Why, then, did they always seem so isolated and remote? They did not work or play together. They lived in worlds apart from each other and from us. Estrangement and nonparticipation were in the air.

Some seemed content to see improvement even within these isolated worlds, particularly if the patient developed a facility with analytic concepts. Some felt reassured if they could but come to an understanding of their patients that made analytic sense. We might have attended more to the fact that Freud had shrunk from the "narcissistic neuroses," leaving a virgin field, or to the fact that many of these patients had already experienced interminable and unsuccessful analyses before coming to the hospital. Finally, however, we did come to see that we needed more than a "properly run" hospital in which analytically oriented psychotherapy alone would do the job of curing schizophrenia.

At any rate, our world and that of our patients ought to coincide more, or surely the improvement we thought we saw was merely our wish-fulfilling illusion. The alienation we saw seemed to be a dynamic process which could go either way under little-known influences. The closer we observed it the less it appeared to be the symptom of a purely intrapsychic process, but rather a product of psychosocial forces. Schematically we saw it thus. At some stage in the patient's life pathologic interaction had begun between him and others in his social environment. Growing estrangement had resulted, which in turn had caused in a susceptible individual a loss of the sense of reality. At some later stage conversion into the secondary symptomatology of hallucinations and delusions was likely. The final state of complete withdrawal with which we were clinically so familiar must be the end product. As it was recurrent and not merely an isolated past event, this process could be studied and affected directly in a properly designed hospital. Inevitably, the dynamics of this present state of fluctuating alienation should command more of our attention than the reconstruction of past events. We could trace in vivo the development of abnormal mental states in their various stages. Thus oriented, we knew that a different approach would be required to reverse the process and to reconcile our worlds. Closeting ourselves with the hospitalized patient in private sessions no longer seemed enough. Often he lapsed into a concreteness of thought which made this approach seem useless. One could appreciate his predicament, split off from society and facing a fearsome chasm. As the breach between him and others widened, contact with reality diminished. Reality was a thing to be shared with others, or it was lost.

When the sense of reality waned, the profusion of secondary symptoms appeared. Some understood these as purposeful mental mechanisms. Others looked for more specific meanings to illuminate the secret core of the illness. Many of us, less easily

convinced of its relevancy to treatment, put aside such speculation and instead explored more empirical methods. All had had
experience with the many specific therapies. Insulin coma therapy, for example, had been held forth as a definitive treatment
which had a specific effect on the brain and thus modified the
course of schizophrenia. Some of us had questioned the theoretical specificity of this treatment. The favorable responses we saw
might be explained by something present among the conditions
of this treatment, which are, to say the least, charged with
drama. Such questions grew eventually into doubts about the
specificity of any treatment for schizophrenia.

We began to speculate more about the involvement of
patients with each other, with the medical and nonprofessional
staff, and in the hospital's culture; in its goals, values, and
traditions. What seemed of growing importance was not so much
the specific treatment but in what manner, under what conditions, and by whom it was administered. Certain modalities
began to appear to us as being more adjunctive than specific.
Even psychotherapy began to assume an adjunctive aspect. The
spirit of this altered view, then, crept increasingly into our
individual therapy. The active study of our involvement with
each other, and our roles and functions, began to replace large
segments of relatively passive sessions.

We had inevitably become involved in treating patients'
families. But the knowledge gained did not suffice to help the
patient. It was not specific either. However, it did alert us in our
relation to the patient, as we came to see the social pathology of
parent, teacher, and community in their relations to the patient.
In the hospital, then, we sought to expose the patient to quite a
different set of relationships and circumstances—a corrective
experience based on rational social interaction. This meant, of
course, that we had to look into ourselves as much as into our
patients. Our analytic knowledge was of great assistance, but in
a group of varying levels of training and stability, this is not an
easy task. It entails the danger that follows from overzealous
inner inspection to the exclusion of an examination of the external reality, which is more or less the same error involved in any
strict analysis of the psychotic patient. What then seemed more
reasonable and more promising was to erect a healthy social

structure. A professional group is more likely to succeed in reaching agreement in such an endeavor than in reaching an agreement on their inner pathology. Not that we would have you believe that achieving this is an easy matter either.

A recurring analogy intrigued us. It seemed reasonable to think that if conditions in a family were optimal—which is to say, fairly healthy—a child reared in such a family could not help being healthy. All our experiences seemed to point in this direction. If true, it would necessarily follow that such a child would hardly ever be in need of any specific psychologic treatment. Likewise, then, in the hospital treatment of mental disorders it was conceivable that the establishment of optimal conditions alone could be sufficient to generate healthier patterns of living and remedy pathology. Specific and individualized forms of therapy might then be either superfluous or simply adjunctive. A community thus formed might promote not only healing but healthy growth and maturation. It would then have the attributes not merely of a therapeutic community, but even, in the absence of formal psychotherapy, a psychotherapeutic community.

Perhaps the patient could learn that he too was playing a role in the process of estrangement. By learning mutual understanding we might hope to bridge the gulf between our separate worlds. Certain conditions might favor this. Did we need to alter ourselves completely to win him over? Certainly we had to be significantly different from others he had known. But to what extent? We knew well that patients constantly pose an insistent demand that we accept this or that piece of unreality and that they are nearly implacable when, in better judgment, we must refuse. Should the character of the hospital reflect to a greater extent the personalities of the ill, or the well, and who is to make the distinction? As we possessed a better grasp of reality, it followed that we should have to take responsibility for establishing conditions based on this knowledge.

Social reality is to a large extent demonstrable and communicable. Instead of merely interpreting reality, we felt that we could represent reality to patients. By doing this clearly, honestly, and consistently, we could hope to induce them to share reality with us. It would not be therapeutic to compromise our own sense of reality merely to accommodate to sick patterns of thought. Certainly we could induce the patient to recognize and accept this and certainly this could be therapeutic. A measure of preservation of our separate identities seems indispensable to the development of healthy individuation in remedial, as well as, normal growth and development.

In remissive phases the grosser forms of estrangement were seen to subside. Yet alienation tended subtly to persist in altered form. As blatant distortions of reality gave way, they were almost always replaced by less obvious expressions of unrealism in the form of problems with authority. Those who administer the conditions of a psychotherapeutic community ought neither abandon what authority seems realistic and appropriate nor react to its challenge with alienating defenses. For we have seen that under optimal psychosocial conditions even the most intractable symptoms may be surrendered. Most ill people are only too ready to yield their unique and isolated positions and the unrealistic attitudes which accompany them if the conditions of their social environment are conducive to participation, representative of reality, and as devoid as possible of alienating reactions. Implicit in our theme is the belief that in the hospital treatment of schizophrenia the very environment must be considered a therapeutic instrument. This is not to say that we would consider any hospital environment as such. On the contrary, it would need to incorporate various essential elements to qualify for the role.

There are various conditions in psychiatric hospitals which in themselves are psychotherapeutic. Hospitals vary in character just as families do, and the principles and practices which give them identity cover a wide range. Whereas the goals of some are limited, immediate, and easily achieved, the goals of others are broad, distant, and difficult to achieve. Some emphasize a psychologic, and some a somatic, approach. Whatever the basic orientation, innumerable conditions are ordinarily incorporated by chance or by design into any residential treatment program. These conditions are significant since they determine either the form or extent of the treatment effort, or both. Although it is not possible to evaluate with certainty the effect of every variable, a few generalizations may be made. The state of health of a hospital determines its therapeutic worth. It has been shown that a hospital can sicken and die and that such an event will be attended by a worsening of its patients. Naturally, we who administer the hospital need to know what is healthy and what is not, both in our patients and in ourselves, and we must act upon such distinctions without equivocation.

In the spirit of exchanging experiences and ideas we wish to enumerate and discuss some of those attributes of the social structure of our own hospital which we believe contribute to its state of health and thereby make it a therapeutic instrument in itself. In the historical progression of thought in psychiatry, attention was necessarily directed at first to individual pathology and much later to the family where it was generated, and finally to conditions in the community where it must be treated. The focus of our attention has turned increasingly toward the latter. We sensed a need to develop as clear a comprehension of the hospital community's reaction to the patient as of the patient's reaction to the hospital community. Therefore, we shifted the emphasis from analyzing the pathology of the hospitalized patient exclusively, as had been traditional, to analyzing and monitoring the hospital's social structure, including the psychology of those engaged in the patient's treatment. This shift in emphasis constitutes one condition which, in itself, has therapeutic implications.

A total underlying commitment by those involved in the hospital treatment of schizophrenic patients is another condition which determines whether the hospital is a therapeutic instrument or not. Scientific curiosity, as well as psychotherapeutic intent, must also be a part of the atmosphere of such an institution. Research should be done there. We ourselves emphasize the "totality of commitment" to the patient as essential to this curiosity and intent. Only the most compellingly realistic considerations are allowed to limit the treatment effort. It is a principle of ours to make maximum use of each treatment opportunity, not to squander it. The histories of patients abound in abortive therapies and lost opportunities. Such indecisive efforts, while superficially conservative, are ultimately wasteful.

Another principle commits one to seek increments of improvement rather than cures alone. We emphasize that the value of any increment, no matter how small, ought not be measured by the efforts spent in producing it. This is quite in accord with the medical tradition that no effort be spared to alleviate illness and that a patient simply may not be forsaken because he does not improve sufficiently to suit us. Unfortunately, economic factors too often dictate the course of therapy. Ideally, such considerations should have no place in a purely scientific formulation of treatment conditions. Nevertheless they do, and their effect on one's commitment must always be kept in mind. Some treatment concepts, born of "economic necessity," are merely forms of abandonment which propel a patient endlessly between home and hospital, from hospital to hospital, ultimately to purely custodial care. Society must beware of developing more sophisticated and less obvious ways of forsaking troublesome and frustrating patients by passing them around in programs which sidestep rather than confront their illness. In other words, our psychologic problems in establishing the ideal conditions of hospital treatment stand forth prominently. Somewhere, for the scientific purpose of establishing the upper limits of potential in the treatment of schizophrenia, as well as for purely humanistic purposes, there ought to be preserved a paradigm of the maximum hospital treatment effort as distinguished from the expedient one.

In our hospital the nature of the goals of treatment itself contributes to the hospital's quality as a therapeutic instrument and becomes incorporated in its character. Over and above the immediate goal of symptomatic improvement and fundamental to a vision of durable gain are broader goals such as these: first, the understanding and acceptance of individual differences implicit in the roles of others; second, the formulation and acceptance of a realistic role for oneself; third, productive immersion in the psychotherapeutic community and identification with it; and fourth, a sense of mutuality and cooperation for the greater good. Needless to say, lesser goals reflect an easier, though not a healthier, way.

The nature of the roles its people play constitutes another condition which determines whether a hospital in itself is therapeutic. We have deemed it neither expedient nor reflective of reality to disown traditional roles, though we have always sought to modify them in healthy directions. Instead, we adopted an attitude of expectation that, without any compromising of roles, there could be mutual acceptance of one another in the hospital by all its participants. Primarily the patient was to be helped with his difficulties. Some preservation of traditional role concepts seemed necessary for interaction to be meaningful. We shunned anonymity in favor of the clear-cut individuation of persons, doctors being unequivocally doctors, nurses nurses, and patients patients. We had no conviction that to act in disregard of the realities implicit in these roles could be in any way therapeutic. It is natural for a significant degree of differentiation to exist in all human relationships which achieve and preserve a sense of individuality. We feel that this is a healthy condition and avoid any undue beclouding of roles for the purpose of establishing a dubious equality. Patients seem to be made uncomfortable by this, for it demeans their role and only makes it more difficult. Treatment personnel do not like obscure role-definition either, as this introduces confusion about responsibility. Instead, we have found that a forthright maintenance of roles is quite acceptable and more comfortable for all. One and all are able to attain better and more realistic views of themselves, achieve deeper mutual respect, and work together more rationally. The job one has to do becomes clearer. The social structure also gains stability and is not so susceptible to idle change. There is a clear need, however, for a constant effort to modify all roles toward healthier perfection.

For example, there is a tendency in some persons to go to extremes, either to get rigidly stereotyped in their roles or to attempt to relinquish them completely. Both are defenses against responsibility for others, and as such are unhealthy and antitherapeutic. At one extreme we may have the stereotype of an insecure and therefore rigid head nurse, a martinet. Her patients have to perform for her like perfect automatons to make her look good in her role. They dare not be sick. She will not take kindly to a soiled schizophrenic youngster with matted hair, and she may get others to imitate her rejection of him. At the other extreme we have an insecure and unassertive doctor who handles his authority like a hot potato, doing all he can to dissociate himself from the role into which his medical responsibilities cast him. He cannot write an order which curtails the potentially dangerous acting out of his patients, for among other things, he is afraid of their reaction against him. Someone else has to do it for him, while he busies himself and others with all sorts of rationalizations about the situation. Each of these, the doctor and the nurse, has avoided responsibility for rendering care appropriate to his role.

It is for the professional team to spot these things and help its members to see what is happening and why, and also to help clarify and support each one's therapeutic role. Roles are plastic. They can be forged and shaped as indicated within the hospital community. In this milieu a good psychiatric nurse can be made of an indifferent or inexperienced one, and a good psychiatrist out of a neophyte. The milieu which can do this has an essential psychotherapeutic condition, namely this: it is capable of healing itself of its own pathology. A hospital ought to be so geared that whenever role abuses are detected, remedial forces can come quickly into play.

We have stressed a sound system and spirit of communication within our hospital as another condition of the psychotherapeutic hospital. The dissemination of information is hardly likely to occur without conscious effort. Healthy people spend much of their time communicating. To seek out and tell another person something, to share a piece of information, is important. More important than what is being communicated may be that there exists a healthy spirit of communication, a condition which marks a healthy society. It is this condition which has most prominently disintegrated in the patient's state of estrangement. What may be really therapeutic in individual psychotherapy is simply that two people get together regularly to share their thoughts, this fact alone outweighing the value of the "interpretations" which may be made at that time. To share flashes of recognition with another, then later to share larger states of consciousness including motivation, is to be involved in the kind of reconciliation on which the growth of a healthy mental state may be based.

Nothing seems to contribute more to the alien state of isolation than not to be "in the know." For harmonious cooperation to exist between people, it would seem essential that they be mutually quite well informed. Things done without the knowledge, if not the consent, of all are likely to breed estrangement, whereas policies openly reached reflect a greater sense of healthy mutuality. We have long observed that coercive purposes may be served by the conscious or unconscious withholding of information, whether from patients or from colleagues.

Discovery of the external world, just as much as of the internal, seems an important factor in the development of a healthy state of mind in a maturing individual. Normal psychologic growth and development must feature an endless series of such discoveries. If they are accurate and complete they lead to a mental state of realism; if not, there is room left for all the pathologic and fragmented conjecture which goes to make up the interior world of schizophrenia, so alien to reality. The healthy operation of a process of discovery can bring about dramatic reversals of trends toward estrangement. We make greater headway perhaps not so much by helping patients to interpret reality as by setting up conditions which will facilitate their own systematic discovery of it. Communication at all levels and the learning which results seem vital in this process. It is probably of equal if not greater importance that the patient, in some areas at least, know as much about us as we know about him. If this is so, no such learning opportunity should be lost to him. If the correct state of communication brings us all to a meeting of the minds, as we think it does, then it must be ranked high among the conditions of treatment which are in themselves therapeutic. This means a great deal of attention must be paid to the mechanics as well as the spirit of it, and equally important, to the exploration of whatever reasons we might have for being less than candid with each other.

Proper professional teamwork is a further condition essential to our hospital as a therapeutic instrument. Even in its presence, sequestration of patient and therapist is a likely occurrence in the treatment of schizophrenia when the exclusive emphasis is on "individual psychotherapy." This may be considered a pathologic development which, in the name of psychotherapy, has the effect of hiding what takes place between patient and doctor. No doubt this is the unconscious purpose of such behavior. Not only has this been seen within our hospital, but also rather surprising pathologic relationships between previous psychiatrists and their patients have come to light after hospitalization. Should these persist within the hospital, they comprise a major impediment to the patient's engagement in its program. A few relationships have been so bizarre as to warrant the appellation folie à deux. More commonly, however, such relationships represent covert abuses of the guiding principle that members of the therapeutic team engage in their transactions with the advice and consent of the others.

Often a patient so involved has been induced to make a show of progress in consideration of privileges and approval according to a kind of "bargain" his therapist has made with him. However, because he has not actually made sound progress, he is set back when thrust into situations for which he really is ill prepared. Unconsciously conspiratorial bargains such as these reflect a spurious form of cooperation and evidence a form of resistance. They serve to alienate patient and doctor from the whole group and its aims.

Likewise, unhealthy effects on patients are seen to result from unhealthy rivalries among hospital therapists. Competition occurs among them to "cure" their patients. The unavoidable outcome is blindness to the objective realities of the patient's illness. A distorted picture of the patient's "improvement" emerges, serving only to insulate him from the therapeutic influence of an informed psychiatric team. One so involved finds himself shielding his patient from the appropriate reactions of a more objective medical group. Similar rivalry is often seen between the various disciplines as well. The destructive effect of this upon the health of the community and ultimately upon that of the patients is unquestionable. It may not be resolved in a psychotherapeutic community by elevating all to equal status as therapists. To do this in our hospital, at any rate, would be to invite chaos.

Just as the team safeguards the patient's progress from the varied personality problems of its individual members, so does it safeguard its therapeutic program from the disintegrative pressures of the schizophrenic society. Anyone who has had prolonged and intensive involvement with such very ill people and their families knows that they may impose stresses upon an individual which become nearly unendurable. These stresses are

in direct proportion to one's depth of involvement. When necessary, a well-functioning team stands as a therapeutic bulwark
which distributes the stress of rampant pathology and protects
against the erosion of healthy forces. It forestalls the development of defensive distancing devices among a vulnerable staff
which would lead only to alienation from patients.

Nothing so reveals a therapist's mettle as his having to
function in a team which takes responsibility for both administrative and therapeutic details without distinction. Here, by
common consent, each member regularly exposes all his transactions with patients to full view. His administrative and therapeutic skills, his strengths and weaknesses, stand revealed. He
must face, before others, whether he is indeed exerting a healthy
influence on his patients. Often he then sees himself either to be
allied in some manifestation of illness with his patient, champi-
oning a pathologic cause they share at the expense of therapeutic
goals, or exploiting the patient for private pathologic purposes of
which he may have been unaware.

Difficult at best to describe, here are some of the more
discernible attributes of our particular team at High Point Hospital. All individual efforts are subordinate, and the activities of
any member with his patients are in daily review. The consensus
prevails when there are differences and the individual therapist
may be thereby overruled. Thus the team-patient relationship
takes precedence over even the doctor-patient relationship, the
team having the power to terminate the latter by reassignment of
the patient to another therapist. Although multidisciplinary, ultimate responsibility is vested in its medical members. There is a
medical leader who retains responsibility but delegates authority. It is essentially hierarchical in conception and function.
Most characteristic perhaps is that the medical leaders of the
team assume the responsibility for making judicious and knowledgeable distinctions between what is healthy and unhealthy.
They assume that this is the particular area of their diagnostic
and analytic competence. They seek to expose pathology in all
quarters, and having made such judgment, to limit, correct, or
otherwise so influence it as to promote the general psychologic
health of the hospital community and its individuals. Here irres-
olution or equivocation are likely to reveal one's own occasional

problems with reality. In addition, the team formulates the policies of our hospital and administers and preserves them. It is both author and custodian of policy and tradition. It has the responsibility for establishing psychotherapeutic conditions and for acting as the rational representative of the healthy social structure. Thus the existence of such a team is a psychotherapeutic condition in itself.

The presence of an analytic orientation on the part of the professional team of our hospital as a therapeutic instrument is the final important condition which we shall touch on. Undoubtedly there are many more. Analysts involved in adapting their methods to the hospital treatment of schizophrenia are required to make an unusual commitment of self. The analyst has been selected and trained to look into his reactions minutely and objectively so as to insure that he will understand them as fully as possible and not allow them to contaminate treatment. He has committed himself to lengthy preparation to secure this ability. In the unusual situations which confront him, his goal is to prevent his biases from ruling his effect on a patient or using for his own purposes another human who has placed himself in his hands. It is precisely here that he has made a bond with himself and with others of similar persuasion to analyze intensively all such relationships in order to avoid the exercise of any such exploitative inclinations, thus putting himself entirely in the service of therapeutic goals. This is not to imply that other men of integrity who are psychiatrists do not strive to do likewise. With the analyst, however, it becomes the very essence of his art and study and the rule of his labors. Learning first to do this, he then imparts it in exemplary, as well as didactic, ways to his colleagues, to his students, and to his patients. What they are able to absorb of this goes to form the matrix of cooperation and mutuality among them all. The understanding of countertransference, of all analytic phenomena, has become a primary purpose among us in our hospital—to be sought not merely in the office with a patient, but in all interpersonal transactions within the psychotherapeutic community.

To be sure, there have been some among us in the hospital over the years who could not acquire this viewpoint. They were those who are content to seek objective clinical skills only, deeming it enough to be proficient at these, and disdaining subjectivity. They usually prove to be the least effective among us, generally remaining detached from full participation in group enterprises and solitary and unidentified with our collective purposes. Thus, when the analytic searchlight is focused with equal intensity on therapists, as on patients, it becomes a significant condition of the hospital which is a therapeutic instrument.

Several observations directed us upon our present path. Patients who had decompensated while under the office care of very skilled psychiatrists and analysts were seen to make rapid strides in the hospital although under the psychotherapeutic care of relatively inexperienced resident therapists. Nothing dramatic, such as electroshock therapy, was used either. Although we generally use the "miracle" drugs in larger doses than office practitioners, some of their patients had nevertheless received substantial doses of medication before hospitalization. At times we were tempted to account for such improvement by the fact that the patient had been removed from the "pressures of life" and the noxious relatives. But often the environment of such patients had been previously manipulated, even to the extent of terminating their work or sending them on extended vacations away from relatives, but to no avail. The positive effect of hospitalization with us, therefore, could not be explained on this basis, particularly as our program did not relieve the patient of environmental pressures. On the contrary, it exposed him to social pressures in an attempt to evoke and study his psychopathology. We could not help but conclude that there were factors in the social structure of our "program" which made it therapeutic in itself. Our only problem, then, was to identify these in the hope that they could be understood and duplicated elsewhere.

We have tried to say that apart from the specific modalities which we are accustomed to accept as *the* forms of treatment for schizophrenia, the very social design of a hospital may be a therapeutic instrument. Such an environment must have certain conditions in order to function with therapeutic effectiveness. The good results accomplished by hospitals which emphasize very different forms of specific treatment may be explained by the conscious or unwitting establishment of an appropriate social design. We may no longer comfortably think of the hospital as an organization that must be run smoothly—simply that the "specific" forms of treatment may be used to good advantage.

The logic of our position is that "administration" and "therapy" are as inseparable as two sides of the same coin. Proper "administration" closely approaches "therapy," if it is not actually that. Such administration does not merely prepare the ground for effective therapy; it organizes and manages the patient and his environment in a manner that in itself is therapeutic. It constructs a way of life with and for the patient which fosters a therapeutic process. It knows that everything which affects the life of the patient will affect his progress in therapy. Administration, then, in the form of the professional team, learns what will affect the patient's life positively and goes about setting up those conditions to accomplish the desired result. It then brings these conditions to bear on the patient in an orderly and properly timed manner to effect necessary changes in his illness and to alter his orientation to reality. In the process the patient gains insight into his faulty functioning and learns healthy ways of relating to others. The positive in him gains the ascendancy, but, if not present, it may be newly created in his personality.

No single hospital can possibly provide a particular patient, especially with adequate and necessary emphasis, all *the* forms of therapy that would fall under the term "broad-spectrum treatment." This is true for various reasons. No one psychiatrist has learned all of them. Psychiatrists have certain predilections, if not biases, concerning modes of treatment. Some are more adept with one form of therapy than another. No one patient or treatment situation permits the application of the many forms of therapy. The physical plant of the hospital—its location, the number and training background of its psychiatrists and ancillary professionals—all determine the modalities it may use effectively. In turn, these and other factors determine the type of patient a particular hospital will admit and the therapies it will provide him.

We are presenting an approach apparently shorn of traditional theoretical concepts. We have dared or have been compelled to take our lead from our clinical experience as we saw it in the raw and to treat patients as this experience dictated. Having proceeded in this way with no choice but to discard dearly held concepts, we have had to travel uncharted seas. We were forced to see that these were theories erected by others on the foundation of a type of clinical experience entirely different from ours. We had to let our own special experience encourage other concepts that were more appropriate to what we were seeing, hearing, and achieving with the use of radically different techniques. While we cannot lay claim to any startling new theory, we believe that such theory must sooner or later come to all of us, and grow from such different clinical experience. We know, too, that we have not been able to completely divorce ourselves from our own background of dogma. It has likely colored our ideas and hampered a better evaluation of our clinical experience. But then, for all of us in psychiatry, this is yet the beginning of our task in treating schizophrenia.

Chapter 9
A Psychoanalytic Hospital Becomes
a Therapeutic Community

in collaboration with Frank G. D'Elia, M.D.

What are some of the characteristics of a psychotherapeutic hospital that create its therapeutic qualities? Primarily it is a highly complex social structure, administratively designed so that all its processes play an active role in the treatment of psychiatric patients. Basic to its organization is the belief of the administrator and the medical staff that the process of mental illness originates in a noxious environment and therefore may be arrested and reversed in an environment that is in harmony with the patient's real needs.

Such a hospital is composed of many groups or systems, each with its own movement, which may often be in conflict with the movement of other systems. The job of the psychiatrist-administrator is to orchestrate those systems. When he does so successfully, he has created an environment that is in itself a therapeutic system. Naturally, if the psychotherapeutic hospital has any scientific basis, we are able to describe its characteristics rationally and in such a way that they can be duplicated elsewhere.

Let us first admit that when High Point Hospital was young, we did not clearly comprehend the social and clinical phenomena we were witnessing. Both of us have been intimately involved in the creation and administration of our hospital. In 18 years we have seen it grow from a rather simple organization that emphasized analytically oriented psychotherapy into a very complex social structure. Its growth always seemed to be prompted by the relative inadequacy of our currently favored treatment approach.

No matter what additional methods we adopted—drugs, shock treatment, group therapy—none seemed to be doing the job alone. No matter how many activities we added to divert, entertain, or involve patients, there never seemed to be enough. No matter how carefully we treated patients or how patiently we dealt with relatives, we always had to seek more meaningful communication. We could never satisfy ourselves that any single approach led to a satisfactory outcome. Yet patients improved, went into remission, and were discharged. The "therapeutic atmosphere" we thought we detected was gratifying, but somehow not scientifically satisfying as an explanation of our successes. We never were quite sure that we understood what was really happening.

Many times over the years, especially during the earlier years of our existence, we have admitted patients whose prognosis seemed hopeless indeed. Our clinical experience had not shown that any one factor, such as psychotherapy, drugs, or electroshock, or any combination of them, had ever helped such patients. More than once we can recall saying, "I wouldn't give a plugged nickel for this chap's future," only to find that he and many others equally sick responded very well if we gave them time. What is more, many of the patients in our hospital already had received every conceivable treatment in other hospitals before entering our program. And they too responded.

Slowly it began to dawn on us that in trying to respond to every inadequacy in the program, we had not merely added pieces to a jigsaw puzzle but had actually fused processes and programs into one single social structure that was itself operating therapeutically. We began to believe we had created a society that had a positive effect on patients because it permitted them to discover, explore, and overcome their sick ways and learn healthier ways of relating to others—ways that became part of them for the rest of their lives. We began to see that our patients were experiencing basic personality changes. We could help a patient become healthier than he had ever been before. We could actually do a reconstruction job—"bring up" a patient all over again. Sometimes it seemed as if we had actually "raised" a patient for the first time, so amorphously formed had he seemed on admission.

No hospital may be called psychotherapeutic unless it is consciously aware of its values and sensitive and active in applying them. Its value system evolves out of the living experiences its staff members have with patients and is usually created by the medical team. The patients' values will almost always be in opposition to those of the staff. In effect the whole treatment process is aimed at bringing the two extremes into harmony. The hospital deals with people who suffer from "sick" relationships with others. Their clinical symptoms are outgrowths of their warped relationships and tend to disappear as patients become able to relate healthily with others. At their worst, patients demonstrate poor judgment and are unable to face and deal with reality; they cannot fulfill their potential with satisfaction, nor can they consistently live by socially acceptable values.

Clearly a psychotherapeutic hospital like ours is by no means a simple structure. It is not a haven where patients can escape their problems; rather it is a social system that permits them to live out and act through their interpersonal problems. One quality of such a hospital is its highly efficient systems of communication, not only between each patient, his doctor, and other staff members, but also among all other professional and nonprofessional personnel. Communication must become synonymous with common understanding, although understanding even among the well, let alone between the well and the sick, is difficult to achieve. The therapeutic process requires patient and therapist to agree upon the goal they are seeking. At the start, each has a different idea of what constitutes health—and a very good thing for the patient that his therapist has a different ultimate goal.

There are many techniques for creating understanding among all staff and patients. They vary from individual psychotherapy to group discussions to patient bull sessions to frequent exchanges between patients and medical staff—the more levels of communication the better. Activities between patients and personnel should be designed to evoke, explore, and overcome the emotional problems that promote the patients' distrust and isolation. Each patient must learn the minutiae of his own personality so that he may begin relating in a healthy manner. For the therapist to contact a patient only in a one-to-one situation is not enough. He must meet him both as an individual and as a member of various groups, on many levels. Those contacts, too, give a therapeutic quality to the whole hospital.

It is important for all professional staff to share a common treatment philosophy in order to give patients the stable environment they need. That is not to say there is no room for exchange of ideas and even disagreement, but at any one time there are limits beyond which disagreement may be antitherapeutic. Mutual understanding and consistency about broad administrative policies, as well as about treatment procedures for an individual patient, are best achieved in regular and frequent meetings of the medical team. True, the individual psychiatrist has the best understanding of his patient and is most sharply aware of how daily decisions will affect him, but when he can come to an agreement with the medical team, he minimizes the possibility of making antitherapeutic decisions. All avenues of communication in the hospital must ultimately lead to the medical team, and all major decisions must emanate from it. If it is to be successful, all members of the medical staff must have a deep investment in the program. Part-time or half-hearted attention is insufficient for its success.

All other personnel who come into meaningful contact with patients must also learn and accept the ultimate goals of the treatment process. Such learning is therapeutic in itself and bears a significant relationship to the experiences of the patients themselves as they learn healthier ways of living.

In the psychotherapeutic hospital the psychiatrist as administrator is the authority on whom all responsibility ultimately falls. He is responsible for dealing with the patients and their critical and taxing demands; with the medical and ancillary staffs and their professional and personal aspirations; with the families of the patients and their assorted anxieties and complaints; with the local and national accrediting bodies and their special demands; with the board of directors and its responsibilities; and with the legal, political, and police authorities who represent society's laws—laws that often conflict with the implementation of the hospital's therapeutic goals, but which must be respected if the hospital is to survive.

Therefore, the administrator must be in the closest contact with all strategic people in the hospital and in the community. He may delegate but never surrender authority. One of his most difficult tasks is to be a strong authority figure without becoming authoritarian or dictatorial.

It is the administrator's task to weld the various disciplines into one therapeutic team, not merely to create an atmosphere in which they may operate independently, each doing his job as he deems best. Only the modification of each discipline, under the guidance of the psychiatrist-administrator, will promote the social structure we are trying to describe. That task is a very delicate one. Each professional staff member will have to sacrifice some part of his image of himself, the aura of his own discipline, and his mode of operating within it. All of them are dear to him, and on them he has based his professional self-esteem. Every professional covertly believes that without him the patient could not possibly have improved to the extent that he has. It is this unconscious attitude that tends to compartmentalize staffs, so that they exist side by side as departments instead of being truly integrated.

It goes without saying that the administrator in the psychotherapeutic-community hospital must be medically trained. He must be conversant with the strengths, weaknesses, and foibles of his medical colleagues if he is to earn their respect. He should be able to teach them, willing to learn from them, and knowledgeable enough to know when to accede to them as a group. He should be a member, as well as the acknowledged leader, of the medical team.

He should be psychoanalytically trained, so that he understands the analytically oriented treatment processes. He should have had extensive experience in working with people in other disciplines and be aware of and sympathetic with their ideas and goals. He should have a basically social orientation about the etiology of mental illness and believe that exposure to a healthy environment can reverse the psychotic process. At the same time, he must be familiar with physiological treatments, appreciate their value, and be open to their use.

One other comment: like all other hospitals, we have been admitting an increasing number of adolescents during the past few years. Today, at any one time, between 35 and 50 percent of our patients are in their teens. They live with our adult patients, receive similar treatments, and are exposed to the same environment. Not only do we also achieve results with them, but they give us no more difficulty than do the adults, although their problems cover the full spectrum of illnesses that adolescents present. Again, we can only conclude that our hospital as a therapeutic instrument has led to these successful results.

We have certain advantages not shared by many hospitals. We are small, with 45 resident patients; compact; and highly staffed. Many patients have no deadlines caused by financial problems and can remain in the program as long as it is helping them. Thus rather than try for a quick, symptom-free result, we can afford to emphasize personality growth and maturity. Our medical personnel, too, seek and experience maturation and thus become better therapists. Our experience allows us to maintain an optimistic approach, although it is tempered by a realistic appraisal of each patient's likely outcome. The psychotherapeutic hospital is a self-improving system, which involves everyone, personnel and patients alike, in its processes.

Chapter 10
Family Therapy in the Hospital Setting

There are a number of ideas and beliefs we have gleaned from our own hospital experience with family therapy which I would like to enumerate. First, we believe in, practice, and encourage the employment of family therapy because it offers a rich opportunity to expand our knowledge of psychopathology and to improve our effectiveness with patients. Second, we believe that it is especially useful in the treatment of the hospitalized patient. Third, we recommend that all of us maintain an open mind with regard to techniques and ideas of what exactly comprises family therapy. Fourth, we believe that in the hospital situation, emphasis should continue to be placed on the primary patient in the very process of family therapy. It is most difficult to get a family to accept the fact that it, rather than the patient, is sick, when the patient is the one in the hospital. We can see, however, that this would be easier when dealing with an ambulatory patient's family. Fifth, we believe that family therapy be most widely used for research purposes. Sixth, we remember that family members also function subject to forces outside the family and that these may be every bit as powerful in affecting the individual as those within the family. This is to say that the wider community, as well as the family, may be regarded as the cradle of mental illness. The family may only mirror and reinforce these injurious pressures, or minimally counteract them. Seventh, we feel, despite our belief in family therapy, that room should be left for the possibility that biochemical imbalances may yet be found to be the cause of mental illness. Eighth, it is urgent that we think of ourselves as primarily medical and psychiatric clinicians, not social scientists, when we engage in family therapy. Essentially we are treating people, not studying social forces per se. In this connection, I would say that family therapy requires an even greater clinical skill than does individual therapy, and a greater ability to make accurate observations, to evaluate more complex psychopathological relationships, and to select and apply correct treatment methods. Ninth, family therapy should be seen in perspective as but one part of our armamentarium, and not as some panacea without which no success with patients is possible.

There is one aspect of family therapy beyond the usual which I want to highlight. We ourselves have concentrated on how the family conducts itself and operates in relation to the "hospital" and the patient's therapist, as well as to the patient. We study and explore for and with him the manner in which he positions himself with us, and do likewise for the way we relate to him. This has to do with matters ranging from visiting hours and calling times to the payment of fees, the so-called administrative aspects of hospital psychiatry. We have concentrated on these dynamics and their pathology as reflections of what has transpired and continues in the family. We see ourselves as having immediately "joined" the family upon the patient's admission to our care.

We believe that pathological relationships within a family may cause mental illness in one or more of its members. By the same token I think there is merit in the idea that an originally decompensating member may trigger off unhealthy responses from other family members. Accordingly, changing him will make these responses unnecessary and cause their replacement by healthier ones. This is our rationale for seeking basic character change in the patient, as well as in the family, rather than mere symptom alleviation.

Pursuant to this line of reasoning, we are sympathetic of the relative's fumbling efforts to contend with the patient's pathology. We do not see these responses necessarily as evidence of pathology, and we do not expect that they should really know better. Unfortunately, most relatives believe that they know how to handle the patient better. In fact, in the face of their failure to do so, they will be self-condemnatory and often doubt their own sanity. Criticism by us only adds to their self-doubt. We are fortified in this approach by our awareness that even the skilled professional has problems dealing with a patient, except that with him we label it "countertransference."

Relatives convey first hand, to him who would experience it, the attitudes and value systems with which the patient was reared. They exude the atmosphere and conflict in which the patient was raised and with which he had to contend. They show us their pathology, thereby making the patient's illness more understandable. At other times they show a relatively healthy situation so that the patient's lack of compensation is not readily fathomed. Occasionally we wonder whether we embarked on family therapy as a defensive reaction because we were constantly subjected to the family's obvious distress and often to their criticism and "unwarranted" hostility. In our type of practice we could not avoid them. The alternative was to shut them out, and the patient with them. Relatives, however, were on our doorstep because they lived nearby, or not at great distances. They paid the bills and had a certain power over the patient, if not over the success of our efforts. If we couldn't lick them we had to join them, or get them to join us in what seemed to be our common goal—the cure of the patient.

Initially we needed the realtive's help to understand and alleviate the patient's acute condition. Unlimited time was not at our disposal. Ultimately we "needed" the family's understanding and acceptance of what, how, and why we were doing things; that is, we needed their trust so that we could do the job we held essential to the patient's welfare. The process of working with them in this manner finally led to a more sophisticated form of family therapy because the family's resistance became evident as the patient faltered or even improved. It became common to hear complaints that fees were too high or requests to release the patient because funds were running low. Petty fault-finding, rejection of instructions, acting out with the patient on visits, and outbursts of unprovoked hostility were other evidences of an unhealthy situation. As a patient changed, family members might become anxious and show hostility toward the patient or us, and misinterpret what we saw to be improvement as "sicker behavior."

On the basis of such repeated experience we recast our thinking and faced the necessity of actually treating the significant relative either individually or in conjoint sessions. In this way we prevented patients from being shortchanged and helped them to understand the relative sufficiently to deal with him. They learned new ways of relating to family even while in the hospital and were supported and fortified by individual therapy too. Also in this manner, we began to furnish significant insights to both patient and family; beyond that, we established an active, many-faceted relationship between the patient's therapist, the hospital, and the relative. The "administrative" aspect of the patient's treatment was also in the therapist's hands. Basically, then, there was much room for an emotionally laden interchange between therapist and relative, both apart from and within conjoint sessions. This left much room for "working through." Incidentally, it gave our staff a unique training experience from which the logic of family therapy became increasingly evident.

Relatives will often "distrust" and experience hostility toward the patient's therapist. They fear showing it to him, for he holds the fate of the patient in his hands. Their feelings, then, are displaced onto "the hospital." The therapist, if not alert and particularly if he has "a problem" relating to the institution, falls in with this hostility. The patient's program set up by the hospital "as a team" then suffers. The patient is caught in the middle. However, this time we see from our living experience with the family, both within the family sessions and apart from them, that this is more or less exactly what happened many times before, and ultimately work it out with the patient and family. This "working out" is possible only because of the way we as psychiatrists relate ourselves dynamically to the family. In other words, we as a group of therapists (that is, a hospital) consciously relate ourselves to the members of the patient's family so as to permit a working through, a gathering of insight on everybody's part, and thereby a healthy alteration in the patient's and the family's psychopathology. This is accomplished in individual work with the patient and additionally in working with the family, both apart from and in conjoint sessions with the patient.

We also tend to regard as family therapy the conscious manner in which we "manage" the family as we work out the patient's therapeutic program. Just as "management" of the patient leads to insight and progress, so the management of the family in relation to the patient and to us as a hospital also leads to insight about the nature of the relative's relation to the patient. For instance, a mother in a symbiotic relation to a son may be forbidden visiting privileges for a long time. In this period the patient progresses and the mother finds that her son can survive without her "help." She is supported by psychotherapy, learns to accept that she is not so critically important to his welfare, that he does not really need her to survive, and accordingly that she need not feel guilty if he does not do well.

After a long separation some relatives will report feeling much better. On occasion a spouse may reevaluate his or her feelings toward the mate and seek an end to the marriage. Had he been permitted to see the patient he could not have extricated himself. Such decisions can then be worked out with the patient in conjoint sessions. Here again, the hospital's management of the relationship is part of the family therapy.

There are several things implicit in the concept of family therapy. One, of course, is that the family is pathological and that other members are also sick, or at least have contributed to the origins and now the perpetuation of the patient's illness. Additionally, however, the concept suggests that family members are potentially useful to the family and the patient. The realization of this in itself may contribute to their well-being. The family now is no longer a helpless outsider, an outcast, the bête noire, but a partner in the therapeutic process. Bearing responsibility, the relative may see the enormity of the task as he himself fails and fumbles. The experience permits him to really grasp the gravity of the illness, the pitfalls in the path, and the human failings of all who are involved. He discovers that no one person is at fault—not he, not the therapist, not the patient—and by the same token, that no one person offers the entire solution. This alone will dissipate a great deal of anxiety and feeling of guilt.

But which comes first—the family's pathology or the patient's? May we not imagine one member of an initially healthy family decompensating first for reasons essentially unrelated to the family? The response of the others as they seek to reestablish the family's equilibrium may be so unsuccessful as to earn our label "sick family." In other words, the originally sick one is the cause of the family's "illness," not the other way around. This is not to say that the family as a whole should not be treated. However, it would seem that the emphasis in the treatment process should be placed differently, depending on one's original proposition. To be sure, there is often more than one actively sick member of a family, and there are often "families" that are sick in the sense that they are not functioning happily and productively. This, however, does not prove that the presence of a sick member actually means an originally sick family. Their responses may be crude and injurious, rather than reparative, but they do not necessarily spring from "sick" thinking and motivation. Unless they do, they should not be considered "sick."

The tendency which exists among some psychiatrists to be unduly critical of the members of a family is often evidence of countertransference. The skilled psychiatrist himself often makes errors even though he spends very little living time with the patient. The family member who must live with the psychotic person constantly has a tremendous handicap and is bound to make many normal errors out of frustration, lack of understanding, and hostility, particularly when he does not realize that the other is sick. His reactions to the aberrant one, no matter how unintentionally injurious, are not necessarily sick unless their origins are unhealthy.

Experience with family therapy would seem to require us to rethink theories and beliefs which have arisen from the one-to-one psychoanalytic model. Some of this has been in process as a result of our experience with group therapy and the therapeutic milieu structures of hospitals. However, the socially oriented psychiatrist has no more proof of the causation of mental disorders than does the organically oriented psychiatrist who believes their origins lie in biochemical imbalances and constitutional deficiencies. The inclination of the first is to study social forces in relation to psychiatric illness and its alleviation. The inclination of the latter is to study physiologic disequilibria and their restoration. The former would logically arrive at family therapy as a means of knowing interpersonal and intergroup forces which distort people, and seek their correction. They have a tremendous task, however, convincing even colleagues who think dynamically, for many cannot see the value of working in any way other than the one-to-one relationship.

Our own experience leads us to believe that "family therapy" as such is a response to the needs of the patient, the family, the psychiatrist, and the "hospital." The fact that families held the power to stop a patient's treatment made it essential that we "treat with" them for the patient's sake. Naturally, this initial benefit for the patient was expanded by the assistance the family and hospital received from the innovation. The needs of the hostile, anxious, and guilt-ridden family members were answered by the process of family therapy. This too was expanded as time went on by some resolution of the family's psychopathology. The essential professional needs of the therapist were initially answered in that he could continue to treat the patient who was in his care. Additionally, he could be relieved of the family's irrational barrage. When the hospital therapist became involved with the patient's pathology he found he needed the family to understand the problems he (the therapist) was having. He needed their cooperation, if not their sympathy. In addition, family therapy answered the therapist's need to have a deeper understanding of the family's "pathology" if he was to gain the professional satisfaction of helping the patient.

All psychiatrists, being human, are subject to their teaching, biases, and experiential background as one-to-one therapists, particularly if they are analytically trained. One who enters into the practice of family therapy must therefore watch against certain tendencies. First, he must guard against overprotecting the primary patient. Second, he must free himself of the tendency to blame parents for the patient's pathology. If he does not, he is bound to be hostile. If he believes that the family as a unit is sick, then it too requires as much understanding, sympathy, and protection as one is accustomed to giving the individual patient. If the patient warrants being taken off the hook, so do the parents to a large extent. They have been and are the victims of other overpowering social teachings; they have also been pressured by their children. Unfortunately I think we as psychiatrists tend to expect too much of them. We tend to blame them for their shortcomings, or consider their injurious behavior as pathologically based, rather than misguided. It would be good for them if they could find some term such as "countertransference" to account for their behavior just as we have to somehow excuse our own culpability when we are less than objective in treating a patient.

Current thinking, to the effect that emotional illness cannot be understood except as an integral part of family illness, tends to minimize individual pathology as an identifiable entity. From the medical point of view this blurs the outlines that aid in diagnosis and direct treatment. It also seems worth determining to what extent any overemphasis on family therapy could be diverting us from improving our techniques of individual therapy. It is conceivable that we might seize upon family therapy to evade facing our frequent failure with individual therapy. To the extent that this might be true, to that extent might an individual therapist be less than thorough with his primary patient.

Family therapy is an effort in the face of our relative failure in treating the mentally ill individual. It is to the good, of this there can be no doubt. However, the trend to focus on the family rather than the individual may be another escape mechanism for us, another subtle way in which we escape the difficult patient himself. Something of this has been true of the rapidity with which we have gone from one form of physical or drug therapy to another in our quest to successfully treat the patient. There have been and are succeeding types of social therapy too—and family therapy is but one such form. To do family therapy, one needs flexibility, stability, tolerance, sensitivity, and the ability to empathize—a combination that is not common in any one person. One needs a confidence in his knowledge of what is actually individual and family health, let alone illness, as well as a trust in the purity of his own value system.

Chapter 11
The Inpatient Treatment of a Child
Drug-Abuser in a Mixed Age Group

in collaboration with the senior author, Guillermo
del Castillo, M.D.

Hospital treatment of the mentally ill has undergone ceaseless modifications, and there have been unbelievable changes from the days when hospitals were little more than dungeons where patients were exhibited to the public for a fee![1]

These changes have been promoted by human zeal and reform movements, increased knowledge of mental illness, advances in technology, and discoveries of psychopharmaceutical agents. Merely confining mental patients in an institution far removed from the active community is now considered obsolete if not deleterious. Instead, active, direct, and dynamic treatment approaches are being used and constantly refined. We now have therapeutic communities, milieu therapy, group therapy, family therapy, after-care facilities, halfway houses, day hospitals and night hospitals. The "open hospital" setting of many state institutions evolved with the effective use of the newer drugs.

Additionally, the trend has been toward a shorter hospital stay and toward the ideal that society should play a role by accepting and rehabilitating the sick upon their return to the community. This trend suggests a minimization of the role of the psychiatric hospital. However, Lewis points out: "It seems more than likely that those who are writing off the psychiatric hospital have not been using it to best advantage. In the past, too much emphasis may have been placed on the protective and

129

custodial aspects of the hospital, to the detriment of an actively therapeutic attitude.''[2]

Although at times irritating and disconcerting, the running controversy over the pros and cons of hospitalization does promote the patient's welfare by fostering better techniques of patient care. Evaluation and reevaluation of therapeutic procedures are indeed necessary. As Lesse observes: ''Nothing is permanent and nothing is all good as far as the health sciences are concerned, and this pertains to psychotherapy just as pointedly as it does to any other branch of medicine or the social sciences.''[3] Skepticism and resistance to innovative proposals are the norm; nevertheless, if we are to make headway, we must abandon archaic customs and traditional theories which have lost application to our present problems.

Changes have been made in response to current challenges, though perhaps not as rapidly as some would like. Whatever the etiology, ever-increasing emotional disorders and drug abuse spotlight the insufficiencies of our health services and their personnel. The growing number of adolescents who clog our services is not due simply to the baby boom of the 1950's. It is more likely due to the fact that our treatment of adolescents is still ill defined, inadequate, and ill prepared to cope with the new era in which practically nobody is willing to suffer in silence.

In reviewing the services for adolescents in New York City, Levy deplores their paucity and suggests reevaluating our concept of treatment when planning for their future development.[4] Specifically, he asks if future mental health programs and facilities could not incorporate adolescents with other age groups. Some institutions have been doing this and the results have been gratifying. Norton, for instance, has listed several advantages for the inpatient treatment of disturbed children, adolescents, and adults when they are housed together.[5] Recently, we presented our own experience at High Point Hospital in the treatment of disturbed adolescents in a mixed setting.[6] Our adolescents, we found, responded as well as adults to a similar program of treatment.

Encouraged by this experience, and with a better knowledge of our hospital as a ''therapeutic instrument,''[7] we were presented with and accepted another challenge—a child who could not be placed elsewhere. Though we did so with a certain degree of trepidation, as when we admitted our first adolescent, we nevertheless admitted this patient into our mixed adult-adolescent population with some measure of hope, if not optimism. The following is a report of our experience with the treatment of a 10-year-old child (decompensated and a hard-drug user) into our mixed adolescent-adult treatment facility.

CASE HISTORY

Billy was 10, Jewish, and a fifth grader in a New York City public school when admitted to High Point. Six weeks previously he had been confined at Bellevue Hospital, where he exhibited a disruptive behavior pattern. He stole the keys to the nursing station, used the phone booths to push drugs, and successfully hid a bag of mescaline and a razor blade in his shoe before he voluntarily gave them up to his therapist. All this was mild compared to his previous behavior. His parents had found him very difficult to control. He often wandered the streets at a very late hour and returned home either drunk from wine or high on marijuana. First his mother, then his father administered beatings in an attempt to discipline him. These did not change his behavior. At one time, in a suicidal gesture, he cut his wrist superficially with a razor blade. His parents, helpless in the face of such incorrigible behavior, finally hospitalized him.

The father, a 34-year-old salesman and habitual marijuana user since age 16, inherited a farm worth $120,000, which he very quickly had to sell to pay his gambling debts. At one time he was arrested for bootlegging and had great difficulty keeping a job. His frequent absences from home caused innumerable quarrels with his wife who suspected him of infidelity.

The mother is a 33-year-old secretary and a marijuana smoker since age 17. She is chronically depressed and has made a suicidal attempt. During 12 years of marriage to Billy's father, she had borne him four children, all boys. Billy is the oldest. A second son died at the age of six months, when Billy was two and a half. The younger siblings are seven and a half and six years of age.

About two years prior to Billy's admission to High Point Hospital, the father left home, presumably "for the last time." The mother then took her children to an apartment where her aging parents were also residing, got a secretarial job, and left her children to the care of her mother. Billy, being the oldest, was often asked by his mother to look after his brothers. At first, Billy took this responsibility willingly and eagerly. He even listened to his mother's tales of woe and tried to console her when she cried to him about his father's absence. Gradually, however, Billy began to shy away from his mother, and began to be irritable, disobedient, and finally defiant. His school work also deteriorated. He did not come home on time and tagged along with the boys in the neighborhood who were twice his age and known to be drug users. He quickly became one of the group and learned to take drugs himself. He sniffed glue, drank wine, smoked pot, took speed, and even snorted heroin. He did not try mainlining because he was afraid of "needles." At this time, he also expressed a desire to have his own apartment and his own mistress!

The mother, aware of what was going on, was nevertheless helpless. Even the presence of the father, who had come home for a reconciliation, did not hamper Billy's activities. The parents, finally fearful that Billy would run afoul of the law, decided to allow him to smoke pot at home, admonishing him to smoke only in the privacy of the home and to abstain from other drugs.

Billy came to the attention of the medical profession about two months before his admission to High Point, when the mother had to be hospitalized with auditory and visual hallucinations. During her two-week confinement, her doctor convinced her to have Billy admitted for evaluation. He arrived at Bellevue Hospital on December 18, 1967 and was transferred to High Point Hospital on January 31, 1968.

On initial interview, Billy gave the impression of being much older than his chronological age. He looked like a 20 year old in miniature. He wore his hair long, sported a turtleneck shirt, tight pants, and boots. He sat quite comfortably and responded to the examiner with very little anxiety. He did complain of being depressed and of taking drugs to get high. He ascribed his depression to his parents' separation two years before. Later on, he denied having any difficulties and complained that "such a big deal" was being made concerning his drug use. He was very proud of this and gladly went into much detail.

He did not want to stay in the hospital but "had to" because his parents wanted him to remain. He would prefer to be home but hates being "mothered," being told what to do, and being "taken advantage of" just because he is small. He feels he is a weakling if he does everything he is asked to do. In the end, he wished he were back in Long Beach where he had lived in a house with his father and mother and brothers, and where he had been very happy "because there I could ride my bike."

DISCUSSION

It is quite evident that Billy's removal from his sick environment was necessary and indicated. At the time of his life when he needs a strong male authority figure with whom to identify, his father leaves home, forcing Billy to assume responsibilities that were anxiety-provoking for his age. These responsibilities pushed him toward his mother, who, instead of diminishing his problems, only added to them by her seductive, helpless, and dependent behavior. This home situation presented a very threatening environment for a growing boy and a dark, unpromising future. The effect in this case was depression, the symptom that Billy complained about. His recourse was to run away from the source of disturbance and make a life for himself in the streets. In his search for security he accepted the company of older boys and young adults who introduced him to their culture. Drugs and alcohol afforded relief.

When the father did come back to assert his authority, it was rather late. His half-hearted attempts were met only with suspicion, fear, and hostility. Billy might not have come to our attention had not the mother herself become seriously ill. At the time Billy was admitted, he presented a front physically and psychologically more consistent with that of a young adult. Underneath, however, he was a youngster who just wanted the chance to be a boy. It seemed to us, then, that our problem was to divest the child of this pathological exterior with which he had

accoutered himself and to replace it with one more appropriate
to his age. Just removing him from his home was not enough.
His symptoms certainly warranted psychiatric treatment in a
hospital setting. The fact that institutions with facilities for child
care had refused him was startling. We naturally speculated at
their justification—that he was too disruptive, and a drug-abuser
who could infect other children with his habit.

PROGRAM OF THE HOSPITAL

At this point a brief description of our hospital treatment
program would seem in order.[8] The hospital houses an average
of some 40 patients who mostly suffer one form of schizophrenic
illness or another, from the borderline to the severe acute or
chronic types. Each patient is seen by an individual therapist
three times a week for a 45-minute session. Psychoactive drugs,
mostly tranquilizers and antidepressants, are used freely as
needed. The hospital is accredited for training and has seven
full-time therapists in addition to several supervising and consulting psychiatrists, all of whom are analytically trained.

One large building houses all the patients and is the scene of
all indoor activities. Patients of both sexes reside in close proximity and commingle in routine activities. Accordingly, the therapist may easily observe the gross behavioral pattern of his and
other patients or have them reported to him in conferences by
nurses and colleagues who also directly observe this behavior.
Consequently there is a highly organized therapeutic structure.
Administrative procedures and policies evolve from the mass of
knowledge derived from a complex of cross-references. Of considerable importance is the fact that much time is spent by the
therapist with significant family members. This practice also
helps to correlate firsthand information and impressions.

The patient population is divided into four groups, in keeping
with their level of behavioral integration rather than diagnosis.
Each group has a different course of activities, depending on its
ability to respect privileges and tolerate responsibilities and
social interactivity. Patients tend to move from the restricted
group to the advanced one, which is an open-floor group with

full privileges. For instance, the more restricted, or Group I patients, are maintained on a restricted program. As improvement occurs, they are moved forward by medical conference recommendation into a variety of communal activities. Supervision by nursing personnel diminishes as the patient progresses through the intervening groups. Finally, in Group IV he may go about the building and grounds more or less as he pleases but is required to participate in a minimum of group activities at assigned times and to assume some of the community responsibilities. This group of patients may visit at home, take educational courses off grounds, and maintain employment in preparation for their eventual departure.

COURSE IN THE HOSPITAL

At the time of Billy's admission, the patient population comprised adolescents and adults in about equal proportion, and he behaved like the 10-year-old child he was. He was inquisitive and curious, fingering light switches and fire extinguishers. He frequently stationed himself at the nursing office and appeared apprehensive of the other patients, who were all trying to befriend him. The following day, however, Billy became his "old" self. He glowed at the attention he received from both patients and staff. He dazzled them with his drug exploits and seemed to enjoy the signs of amazement he elicited. Most of the adolescent patients in the hospital had had some experience with drugs, and having this in common, Billy readily joined this group. This novelty, however, gradually wore off in the ensuing weeks. Patients seemed to tire of listening to him, so Billy began to ingratiate himself in one way or another. Ordinarily he took advantage of the fact that he was the focus of attention.

He was advanced to Group II where his interest in arts and crafts was observed and encouraged. By the second week he was moved ahead to Group III, since the staff wished to provide him with more activities. But this time he began to defy hospital rules and regulations. When caught and reprimanded by an aide, he would insist that another aide had given him permission to do such and such and thus try to evade responsibility. He would lie and turn one aide against another, or else arouse the sympathy of older patients, who then defended him against any reprimand. In individual sessions he used the same denial and blamed others for his predicament.

The staff slowly became aware of the patient's behavior and its effects on patients and nursing staff. The latter began to experience feelings of anger and frustration, and the medical staff then decided on program changes which would be more suitable for Billy and more tolerable for the nursing staff. Accordingly, one female nurse from each shift was assigned sole responsibility for Billy's care and supervision. All communications from the medical staff in the person of the treating psychiatrist were channeled to these nurses. Communications from Billy in the form of complaints or requests were also directed either to these nurses or to Billy's therapist. The nurses assigned to him were carefully coached by the medical staff as the patient's program was formulated.

In essence, the program was designed to curtail any routine or activity which might be inconsistent with his age and status in the hospital community. For instance, his bedtime hour was made an hour and a half earlier than the rest of the patient population; he was allowed only one cup of coffee a day; he received tutoring twice a week with a supervised study period everyday except weekends. In short, we tried to give Billy an atmosphere approximating that of a healthy home situation, with parental authority that was firm but understanding and flexible.

As expected, Billy responded with a great show of anger and tears. He complained bitterly about his regime and affirmed that he could follow the regular routine as well as anyone else, that the program set him apart from the others, and that he did not like the nurses assigned to him. He was told, however, that the staff's decision was fixed and he was to give things a try.

Billy followed the prescribed program but with much sulking and covert rebelliousness. He tried to manipulate as usual, but without his prior success. He did, however, seek out the company of one particular adolescent who was extremely resistive and openly hostile to the hospital. Nevertheless, by the end of the third week his parents both remarked that Billy appeared quite calm and pleasant. Billy's behavior continued to improve, and he became less rebellious and defiant. By the end of the second month of his stay he was actually cooperative and his visiting privileges could be gradually extended until he was able to go off grounds and visit with his brothers.

Quite unexpectedly, in the middle of his third month of stay, Billy ran away from the hospital and had to be brought back against his will. When questioned about this, he claimed that he was angry at the staff for not having given him a longer visiting time. On further inquiry, it came out that he had not really enjoyed his visits, particularly when his parents brought his two brothers with them. He complained that they were too noisy and too active, talking all the time, always asking for things, and making it difficult for him to talk with his mother.

After a few days of restriction, Billy was permitted to resume his former activities. He repeatedly promised not to run away and was very apologetic. At this point, conjoint family therapy sessions were instituted, including his parents and brothers. All had been prepared for this procedure, and we had several things in mind for it. One was to study the family in action and its effect on the patient; the second was to elicit from and explore with them their pathological attitudes for correction; the third was to involve the parents in sharing the responsibility for Billy's care. The father, who had always been passive and irresponsible, was encouraged to assert his authority. One of the first things he told Billy was that he was trying to give up his own marijuana habit. The mother hastened to confirm this and also reassured Billy that she was doing the same.

Up to this point, the parents were still undecided about continuing their marriage or separating. The father wanted more time to think. He claimed that he was just about getting settled in his job and enjoying it. Both were also seen separately from the family sessions and helped to see that if they wanted Billy back they would have to mend their ways and help each other. Failing this, some other arrangement, such as a foster home or boarding school, would seem better for Billy. The patient was not informed of the parents' continuing indecision.

Billy's improvement continued apace as he became decreasingly guarded and hostile. He was increasingly communicative, particularly when the nurse assigned to him was present in sessions. Although his attitude toward his male therapist remained rather cool and reserved, he was less so toward his father. Off-ground visits with the father alone were promoted. They both enjoyed these visits and looked forward to them eagerly. Gradually, the father became increasingly assertive and the mother's role became less prominent. This was apparent also in the conjoint family sessions.

By the fourth month Billy had progressed further in the group system and was assigned to the Arts and Crafts and the Garden Committees. His performance was comparable to that of the older patients, and the individual program that had originally been designed for him became less and less distinct. With very little exception, the regular management program for the bulk of the patients became applicable to Billy as well.

During the fifth month of Billy's stay his parents announced their decision to give their marriage another try. They were also making plans to move back to Long Beach to get away from the drug scene of the city. Both seemed sincere and determined to save their marriage and family. Billy's more extended visiting at home continued to go well. His younger brother, who became increasingly psychotic, was placed in therapy with Billy's referring doctor.

As anticlimax to this narrative, a brief episode took place in the middle of the fifth month. When everything appeared to be under control, Billy suddenly erupted with a violent outburst of anger which was almost psychotic in proportion. The provocation appeared rather slight in comparison to his reaction. What had transpired was caused by a nurse confiscating a book *(Catcher in the Rye)* that Billy's mother had given him. Billy started to scream and accuse everybody of trying to kill him. He carried on for quite a length of time and no amount of verbal reassurance could calm him. He threatened to run away. Because of this his medication had to be doubled (Billy had been on Mellaril, 50 mg. q.i.d. since admission) and his activities curtailed by placing him in a more restricted group. However, after a few days, he regained his control, and the privileges and responsibilities he had lost were restored.

By the sixth month of his stay Billy's behavior had improved to the point where he could be entrusted with greater freedom.

He was placed on the open floor, and his medication was halved. Although we would have preferred Billy to remain longer, his parents' pressing financial difficulties prevented us from going further with his therapy. On August 2, 1968, therefore, he was discharged to the custody of his parents with the recommendation that he continue ambulatory therapy with his referring doctor. At the time of his discharge, Billy's adult artificiality was gone and he was a very happy boy going to his new home. As of this writing (late 1969) Billy's doctor informs us that he is doing well, attending school, and keeping his appointments regularly and on his own.

SUMMARY

The abuse of drugs by adolescents, and more lately by children, has presented psychiatry with a crisis situation. We are in a dilemma and relatively helpless both to understand and to remedy that which has descended upon us with crashing rapidity. Our facilities are meager and still poorly prepared for handling the problem of serious drug abuse by children. We have been geared for a more adult population or young people with emotional and mental disorders uncomplicated by drug abuse and addiction. Our ability to cope is also complicated by our differing beliefs about personality development, diagnosis, and the advisable treatment environment. As though the situation were not complex enough, there is a thick overlay of social, economic, and political considerations which complicate and hamstring our efforts. Further, the general public seems to be much more emotionally involved and insistent on a role than it ever was with the problem of mental illness per se. This seems particularly true as drug abuse increasingly invades the younger segments of our population. Of significance, too, is the sickening impact this crisis has on psychiatrists as individual members of society who react with understandable anxiety and a sense of foreboding.

Though a single patient is involved, this presentation illustrates the gamut of presenting problems when dealing with a drug abuser, particularly a child. First, the difficulty in getting parents to face the problem and accept hospitalization; second, the difficulty of containing the patient in an adequate facility prepared to receive and hold him; third, the obvious paucity of facilities; fourth, the question of the nature of the facility, that is, should it deal exclusively with patients of the same age group or be a mixed patient population? As important as the question of the age of fellow patients seems to be, the nature of the treatment program to which the patient is exposed is of equal significance. Our own particular approach with its many facets is related in some detail. The fact that it met with moderate success provides some measure of optimism. In the face of the crying need for bed space for children, a need that will not be satisfied in the foreseeable future, our experience suggests the feasibility of treating child drug abusers in a mixed age group.

REFERENCES

1. Redlich, F. C., and D. X. Freedman. *The theory and practice of psychiatry.* New York: Basic Books, 1966.
2. Lewis, A. B., Jr. "Effective utilization of the psychiatric hospital." *Journal of the American Medical Association,* 197:871–77 (September 1966).
3. Lesse, S. "Obsolescence in psychotherapy—a psychosocial view." *American Journal of Psychotherapy,* 23:381–95 (July 1969).
4. Levy, A. M. "Services for adolescents in New York City, mental health services for adolescents." *Proceedings of the Second Hillside Hospital Conference.* New York: Praeger, 1968.
5. Norton, A. H. "Evaluation of a psychiatric service for children, adolescents, and adults." *American Journal of Psychiatry,* 123:11 (May 1967).
6. Gralnick, A. "The adolescent inpatient: treatment considerations and report on ninety-two cases compared with ninety-two adults." *Diseases of the Nervous System,* 30:833–42 (December 1969).
7. Gralnick, A. *The psychiatric hospital as a therapeutic instrument.* New York: Brunner-Mazel, 1969.
8. Gralnick, A., and F. D'Elia. "Role of the patient in the therapeutic community: patient participation." *American Journal of Psychotherapy,* 15:63–72 (January 1961).

Chapter 12
A Social Nursing-Therapy Service:
Concept and Development

in collaboration with Frank G. D'Elia, M.D.

There have been two main currents of thought in psychiatry running rather parallel courses. One is based on the belief that mental illness is organic in origin and its treatment primarily physical. The other is embedded in the belief that the beginnings of psychopathology lie in the early history of one's social relationships. Neither theory has led us to the satisfactory control and treatment of psychiatric disease. The second theory owes its main impetus to psychoanalysis, with its emphasis on psychopathology being rooted in the triadic relationship between child and parents; its treatment is entrusted to the dyadic therapist-patient relationship. This treatment model has influenced many hospital programs.

It may be fairly said that the socially oriented theorists have more seriously sought an accommodation with the others and that of the two approaches, it contains the rootlets of social psychiatry. However, social psychiatry has come upon the scene with gathering force for several reasons other than the influence of psychoanalysis. First, the dyadic therapeutic technique leaves too many people unattended. Even its offshoots of group and family therapy have been unable to meet the rising need for providers of service. Second, the massive increase in the number of those sick and those with serious symptoms and habits have compelled us to seek more comprehensive methods of solution. Third, the physiologic treatments have not diminished our problems to any major degree. Fourth, our social scientist colleagues have alerted us to the strong possibility that social conflicts give rise to tensions conducive to mental disorder. They suggest that the way people are socially related produces illness, that if such disorder is to be diminished, the nature of "social relatedness" needs to be changed on a global scale. Fifth, the intra- and international struggles, the violent polarizations of peoples politically, economically, and racially, the presence of poverty and starvation in the midst of plenty, and the constant presence of war in the face of a universal preference for peace and goodwill—all of these contradictions somehow force themselves on even the most organically minded of psychiatrists as at least contributing to the creation of psychoses. It will be said by them that "society is sick," and accordingly, they will be sympathetic to "social psychiatry." Sixth, the introduction of the new value system, that all people have the right to quality care, makes imperative the discovery and use of new concepts and means of implementing them. Social psychiatry has been spawned by this new tradition and will probably shunt aside the very psychoanalytic concepts and techniques which gave it some reason to be.

If nothing else, the immensity of the problem compels our search for solution on a global scale. It is as though we had nowhere else to turn but to the social structure and social relationships, with the hope that in their alteration, we will in some way alleviate the many millions of our mentally ill. Thus "social psychiatry"! It will be variously defined, but most will agree that it rests on the assumption that mental and emotional illnesses arise from or are seriously affected by social disturbance and that they are significantly affected by dramatic changes in the social relationships to which one is exposed. With this as its foundation of thought, High Point Hospital set about to develop a social structure or "hospital family" which would have a healthy effect on patients, that is, that it would undo the effects of the psychotogenic environment. Our task would have been easier if we had known more exactly what conditions produced a healthy person.

Originally our hospital had the traditionally compartmentalized system of medical, nursing, and occupational and recrea-

tional departments, aside from the usual nonprofessional departments. They functioned independently with less-than-complete
communication. Understanding and acceptance of a mutuality of
goals for the patient, as well as joint responsibility for their
fulfillment, left much to be desired. This was not the best team
effort. The major emphasis was on traditional insight therapy,
the search for early traumata, and the patient's motivations in
whatever he did. The nontherapist roles (or departments)
existed merely to make available a necessary atmosphere in
which the insight therapy could have its desired effect. In addition, there was the element of the psychotherapist-administrator
split so prevalent in the analytically oriented hospital.

It did not take us long to see that such an atmosphere was
intangible rather than clearly defined and hardly as conducive to
personality change and growth as we had imagined. Insight was
not enough in an atmosphere which appeared to make it achieva-
ble but which was not necessarily of itself productive of symptom-alleviation, let alone personality change. Such change, or
rehabilitation—which was really what we sought for our inpatients—seemed to need more than an atmosphere. Our task,
then, was to develop this intangible atmosphere (or loosely
compartmentalized operation) into a structured social system.
We first faced changing the nature of the social relationships
between the professional departments, namely the medical,
nursing, occupational, and recreational therapy personnel. As
this developed we increasingly placed our emphasis on learning
about the patients from their participation in the work of committees we established. In other words, as we changed our
professional relationships, we inevitably had to change our relationships to the patients. Social-relatedness changed throughout
the hospital. Originally the very recognition of the requirement
for change set a number of actions and new ideas into motion
almost simultaneously—so much so that it is difficult to know
and describe the order in which they occurred. Our earlier
thinking and actions of the late 1950's are described in three
papers[1,2,3] and our book, *The Psychiatric Hospital as a Therapeutic Instrument.*[4] Our general aim was to imbue everyone with
shared therapeutic attitudes and concepts, so that a "psychotherapeutic consensus" could be achieved.

We had become disenchanted with the notion that every activity of the patient was *therapy* and decreasingly subscribed to the idea that there really were such animals as "occupational," "recreational," "music," and "art" therapy as such, any more than there was "therapy" inherent in the numerous other activities in which hospital patients engaged. Patients participated in many of these activities, as well as productive work, before coming to the hospital, and still became ill. If these activities within the hospital served any therapeutic value, it was not inherent in the occupation or recreation itself but in some aspect of it—perhaps the therapeutic concepts and social comportment of those associated with the patients in the activities. The problem was that these were as yet undefined, unstructured, and unspoken. There seemed to be some analogy to the situation in psychoanalysis. For a long time it seemed that its therapeutic aspect was the insight achieved by the patient in his impersonal relation to the analyst with whom little of any real human contact existed. The analyst was a screen against which the patient played out his infantile neurosis. As analysis matured, however, some began to believe in the power of suggestion and learning in therapy and that actually there was and should be an active human relationship between the patient and the doctor. It came to be thought that it was the interpersonal relationship which contributed to the cure and not the insight about early traumata. Some of this thinking has been developed recently by Thomas.[5]

Similarly, then, in our analytically oriented hospital we sought to discover what social concepts and human interactions could be considered truly therapeutic. If we failed to find such it would be incumbent upon us to establish those factors and conditions which yielded healthy personality growth and change, aside from symptom-alleviation. You may be sure, it was not easy to think in these terms, let alone act on them, to challenge entrenched concepts and discard tried and traditional hospital techniques.

Among the first changes we made in role definition was to alter the isolation of the medical psychotherapists in the dyadic office relationship. They were no longer limited to merely seeing the patient in office therapy three sessions a week, but were called on to participate with groups of patients and share certain functions with them. Concomitantly, they had to surrender the self-inflating notion that they alone cured the patient and that the other professionals were merely window dressing for maintaining a harmonious atmosphere in which they, the therapists, could work their cures undisturbed. Instead they had to work closely with these others in conferences to draw on their assistance and to assign them functions in the therapeutic process. This was not easy for therapists to accept without constant reminding that seven sessions a week would be unsuccessful without good teamwork and administration. In addition, they were called on to work closely with families for their assistance. They were not afforded the luxury and defense against the family which a social worker would ordinarily give. Further, they were not permitted to be split off from administrative responsibilities. Instead, in conference as a team, they made all of the clinical-administrative decisions on patients. The patients knew this, that they were therefore related to more than just their own therapist, as well as being aware that the substance of their sessions was shared in the staff meetings. This way there could be no secrets; the patient was saved from unhealthy countertransference reactions on the part of his therapist by the intercession of the rest of the team. Incidentally, these changes were not foisted on the medical staff, but evolved over a period of several years of conferring and decision-making by staff members. Included in these conferences, of course, were members of the nursing and "occupational-recreational therapy" department. This was true for all the changes we made and describe in this article.

More or less concurrently with the above-described changes, we began to fuse the occupational-recreational therapy departments into one by using a group worker. We called this new unit the *group work department*. Naturally it was brought into close relation with the medical and nursing staffs; here, too, new concepts and attitudes developed. Instead of these departments being separate units as they had been, with patients being shuttled by nurses from one to the other to be "acted upon" by its own members with their own particular expertise, these departments were slowly interdigitated, welded, and amalgamated.

Members of the group work department participated in many of the activities ordinarily considered nursing functions, just as medical therapists participated with patient committees functioning under the aegis of the group work department. Members of the nursing department increasingly participated in the group work department's activities, namely, occupational, recreational, and patient committee work functions. Slowly and surely, the medical, nursing, and group work departments were amalgamated. The terms *occupational* and *recreational therapy* began to disappear from our language, as did the concepts associated with them.

We began to deemphasize the skill aspects of the activities and to highlight their personality-development possibilities and the social skills to be acquired in the interpersonal relationships involved. Thus we turned more to the social substance, rather than the form, of the therapy given. The emphasis was on *work* and all the problems it created for people involved in it, so that these interpersonal conflicts and associated anxieties could be evoked, studied, and overcome. While we did not belittle the personal satisfaction to be derived from a craft well done, it became more important to us to observe and report in staff meetings how such a person reacted. Did he lord it over others less skilled? Did he try things at which he was less apt to be outstanding? Did he help his fellow patient acquire adeptness at his particular skill? Was he a loner? Did he join and cooperate? What was his tolerance point? In other words, were his social relationships healthy, as we conceived such to be?

The tack we were taking was to see the activities as social relationships which could be studied and used to help the patient see himself more as he was and where he needed changing for the better, and with information thus gleaned, to assist the therapist to help the patient along these lines in the therapeutic sessions. It seemed increasingly to us that here was where the therapeutic aspects of these activities lay in the hospital setting, namely, in the conscious exposure of patients to social pressures to elicit their conflicts for solution on their own or with their therapists. In like manner, the very environment constructed contributed to this process without necessitating the intervention of a therapist. Herein lay the core of the idea of the hospital itself as a therapeutic instrument, an institution of relationships beyond the concept of the "therapeutic community."

In the process of making these changes, we were really seeing social psychiatry in birth. Out of these changes in social relatedness,[6] structure, and attitude arose the concept of the social nursing-therapy service and the groping toward its implementation. It was something of a blow to finally see the obvious, what had been staring us squarely in the face for a long time. In psychiatry there was always a nursing department! It was always treating patients, yet was never called a nursing *therapy* department. Why? Was it because the nurse was merely the handmaiden of the doctor, his Florence Nightingale, always there in his shadow to carry out orders, to take the temperature, give the injection, take the pulse or blood pressure? This answer did not seem adequate, especially in the decades of the therapeutic community. Somehow the nurse did not have a therapeutic role, although she spent more time with the patient than anyone else. She sent or took him to the occupational or recreational therapy department or even to the music, art, and poetry therapy departments. But even in the age of social psychiatry, hers was not a therapy department. Quite a contradiction for psychiatry to ponder!

Here we were at High Point Hospital, organized with the members of the nursing department participating in medical staff conferences, making decisions with doctors regarding clinical-administrative matters, and participating in all of the patients' individual and committee activities of the group work department. They did the latter to the point that they could and did run all of these activities in the absence of the group workers and arts and crafts and recreational workers. Thus in our hospital community, psychiatry was being practiced quite differently, technically and theoretically. In fact, it appeared to us that it practiced community psychiatry within its own boundaries because it was an integrated professional and patient community that brought its power and expertise, as such, to bear on the patients therapeutically.

But there remained a problem which at first appeared to be on an administrative and organizational level, but which soon had to be seen as having therapeutic overtones. The director of nursing had certainly risen to a position of significant authority alongside the group work department head and the senior medical authority. Since the concept of social psychiatry as it had developed in our hospital meant that there were therapeutic aspects to all of the patients' social relationships involved in his every activity, who was to have on-the-spot chief authority to resolve the many problems arising from the patients? It would be too much to have each problem brought to the senior medical authority. A choice had to be made between the group work department head and the director of nursing. The choice was made in favor of the director of nursing who had long worked with the patients in groups and as individuals. In addition, when problems involved the physical evaluation of the patient and possibly his life, she was better trained and equipped to make the proper decision and to be more alert to the need for contacting the medical department.

Once this decision was made, the implementation of the concept of the social psychiatric nursing-therapy service had its own logic: the fusion of the nursing and group work departments into the one unit. The director of nursing now has chief authority over all activities, as well as jurisdiction of all the activity therapists to whom she delegates responsibility. In addition to promising to prove a therapeutic advance and congruent with the significance of social psychiatry as such, the design has obvious administrative advantages. It is a moot question how applicable this would be to a larger institution, but in our small organization we are inclined to view our current system as social psychiatry in action in a hospital setting. The emerging relationship of the newly designed nursing-therapy service to the medical staff is already proving both of interest and challenging.

SUMMARY AND THEORETICAL FORMULATION

In the foregoing we have described our unique hospital clinical experience, an organizational restructuring of an institution, and the reordering of the relationship of its social groups. All of these have encouraged, if not compelled, an examination and reassessment of the theories to which we ordinarily cling and use to explain clinical findings. We have changed our emphasis from the forms of therapy to the more important social substance of the interactions between those who people the hospital. As a consequence, there is some logic to our search for other theories to explain the validity of the changes made and the reason they appear to work successfully.

It might be that the consolidation of these social systems, otherwise at variance, made it easier to arrive at a consensus, an understanding and mutuality of goals all of which are of therapeutic value. This, also, to some extent was the administrative-therapeutic rationale for the organizational decrease in the number of social groupings. The fewer the barriers, the easier it is to concentrate on the consensus-forming process and the easier it is to reach agreement. These are factors which are, in themselves, therapeutic.

It is generally thought that the greater the harmony, love, and respect between parents, the more wholesome the child's environment and the healthier he is likely to be. This is considered true, especially among psychoanalysts, though built into their theory is the oedipal complex, which seems to promote almost insoluble child-parent conflict even under the most ideal conditions. The changes we wrought in the standing of the nursing service vis-à-vis the medical staff—giving them a more balanced and important role in relation to the patient—might be seen as having changed an unhealthy family relationship in which the father was chief authority and the mother was relegated to a subordinate position, to a healthier one for the child (patient). By the same reasoning, one can say that the conditions which had previously prevailed would be similarly unhealthy in a family where the mother is domineering and the father is passive and voiceless. This is the condition common in many psychiatric hospitals where the doctor-patient ratio is so poor that the psychiatrist has no time for close patient care and the by far major part is left to the nursing staff. Using the same theoretical base, this type of imbalance would also be considered an unhealthy environment. In the first instance, it is considered similar to a motherless home, and in the second, to a fatherless one.

We may say, then, that in our hospital the condition that had prevailed, namely with the doctors definitely in the ascendancy, had been altered and a more even balance of authority between the paternal and maternal figures achieved. The role barriers between them were lowered, and they could consequently develop better understanding and harmony and more easily reach a psychotherapeutic consensus and establish mutual goals for the child figure—the patient. All of this contributes to the therapeutic environment. The social substance rather than the form of therapy could now be given proper attention. Such conditions were considered infinitely superior to the other conditions and were therefore healthier for the patient. They gave him a better chance to develop a more balanced personality and further his growth as a human being.

This theorization to make what we had done understandable, acceptable, and palatable since it is so technically unorthodox is traditionally correct but not necessarily satisfactory.

What would explain why the two groups seemed to work together more harmoniously and cooperatively when their social relatedness was altered by a diminution of their role differences? All too often, people in such apposition engaged in a power struggle. *Traditional theory* seemed too simple. What would guarantee the continuity of the healthy spirit of these groups and prevent its deterioration? Why in a hospital so structured would a psychotherapeutic consensus arise and a mutuality of goals for the patient be perpetuated?

It would seem that the single, unswerving, purposeful value system of the larger social structure—that is, the hospital— would play a part in keeping its subsystems from clashing. The role and strength of the leaders is important in keeping the hospital's chief goal foremost in mind. Such considerations might spell the difference between what prevails for the patient in our hospital and the child even in an ideal family environment. The family is immersed in a larger system (society) that has contradictory values which may adversely affect and even over- whelm any member of the family. None of its members is immune from the conflicting and negative forces no matter how sound the family may be. The hospital, on the other hand, is a complete social unit, or team, all of whose members are care- fully selected, kept working together, and are educated to and motivated by the same value system. It is not limited to the doctors and nurses alone, but is a society of its own with limited contradictory standards and with goals consistent with its everyday life. Consistency, stability, and obvious concern for the patient are factors which affect personnel as well as patients and stimulate them to maintain mutual goals, cooperation, and the psychotherapeutic consensus.

REFERENCES

1. Gralnick, A., and F. D'Elia. "Role of the patient in the therapeutic community: patient participation." *American Journal of Psychotherapy,* 15:1:63–72 (January 1961).

2. Lind, A., and A. Gralnick. "Integration of the social group worker and psychiatrist in the psychiatric hospital." *International Journal of Social Psychiatry,* 11:1:53–58 (1965).

3. Gralnick, A., and F. D'Elia. "Social forces and patient progress in the psychotherapeutic community." *International Journal of Social Psychiatry,* 14:2 (1968).

4. Gralnick, A., ed. *The psychiatric hospital as a therapeutic instrument.* New York: Brunner-Mazel, 1969.

5. Thomas, A. "Purpose versus consequence in the analysis of behavior." *American Journal of Psychotherapy,* 24:1:49–64 (January 1970).

6. Lennard, H. L., and A. Bernstein, eds. *Patterns in human interaction.* San Francisco: Jossey-Bass, 1969.

Chapter 13
Intensive Inpatient Psychotherapy of Adolescents

Traditional psychoanalytic technique isolated the patient from the therapist as a human being. The modern practitioner brought them together as people engaged in a purposive human relationship within a larger environment. Ultimately there evolved the belief that the treatment of the inpatient, whether with drug or psychotherapy, cannot be isolated from the social structure in which he and those who treat him are immersed and to which they are continually responding. When we see the patient and those treating him as humans inseparably involved in their society, we are bound to consider the effect of one on the other as a human being and the impact of their setting on both. It is similar to the belief that one may have a humanizing effect on the other and that their common hospital society has a humanizing influence on either. Inhospital psychotherapy as a modality, then, cannot be isolated from the environment in which it is practiced, any more than it can be isolated from the people engaged in its process. Essentially one cannot conceptualize, describe, or evaluate psychotherapy without a simultaneous study and integration of the hospital's social structure into the consideration of any aspect of the patient's psychotherapy. As Roy Grinker would put it, they are interpenetrating social systems.

In any psychoanalytic discussion one starts with certain assumptions and beliefs which warrant statement. A psychiatrist's thoughts are the end result of his total life experiences, which include those of his early and later years, up to the very time he puts a pen to paper or mounts a platform to expound his ideas. They are the culmination of a continuing process of acculturation, including his training experience with students, teachers, and analysts and the system of values he adopts during his life. They are affected by the action he is capable of taking to implement these values.

Accordingly, an audience should have some information, no matter how sketchy, about a speaker's background in order to place his remarks in perspective. I was the youngest of five in a lower middle class family which was upwardly mobile until the Depression, at which time I was in my late adolescence. Though my values were the same as those of my family, I seemed to be more venturesome, ready to see and accept challenge, and to favor and participate in change. Though respectful of tradition I always seemed to find myself among those who were, to borrow a later phrase, "doing their thing." I entered training with a group of analysts who had just left the New York Psychoanalytic Society under the leadership of Horney. When they split, I was among the students who went with the teachers who formed the first psychoanalytic faculty of a medical school and was among the four who comprised the first psychoanalytic graduating class of a medical school, that of the New York Medical College. It could not be otherwise but that I would be a charter member of the Society of Medical Psychoanalysts and of the Academy of Psychoanalysis.

You might guess that at that time the analyst I selected was among those then considered most "unorthodox." I recall a session some 30 years ago vividly. As I lay sweating on the couch one summer day, before air conditioning, I expressed my belief that given the condition of mankind working together harmoniously, there was no end to what man could accomplish and that it was my conviction that someday he would actually fly to the moon. I remember the analysts wry retort: "Really?" I never did discover whether he believed it or thought I was daft, for I was only a psychoanalytic student, wholly unversed in matters having to do with aerodynamics and the solar system. Today we are en route to Venus and someday will land there.

My earliest years of training were in a New York state hospital, during which time I was simultaneously in analytic training and directed a shock treatment unit. One type of experience affected the other; I could write about the psychotherapeutic and interpersonal aspects of insulin coma therapy[1] while keeping my psychoanalytic theory and practice in perspective. There followed six years of private psychoanalytic office practice and then the founding and directing, for the past 22 years of a proprietary psychiatric hospital. I helped pioneer in the treatment of adolescents among adults with intensive psychotherapy to the point that ordinarily 50 to 60 percent of our patients now are 21 years old or younger. While at first I treated patients for a considerable period of time, I am now confined to the post of medical director, which includes carrying chief clinical and administrative responsibility. Therefore, I cannot talk as a *therapist* in the strict sense of the word except as administration and supervision of a psychotherapeutic treatment team may be seen as playing a therapeutic role. From my vantage point, however, I can give an overview of our program of intensive individual psychotherapy of the inpatient adolescent in the highly developed social system we call High Point Hospital. I should add that some of our research studies indicate that the qualities of the leader in such a program may very well have an effect on a patient's therapeutic result.[2] At any rate, from the nature of my own hospital experience with the adolescent has come a view of him, his pathology, and a method and theory for his treatment that might be of interest.

I do believe that we in psychiatry and its subbranch, psychoanalysis, have hardly touched the surface of knowledge of those life experiences which affect and determine the nature of our thoughts, feelings, and actions. If anything, our relative impotence alone may be sufficient evidence that we have been and are off on the wrong foot entirely. True, we have elaborated theories, some of them fanciful, to account for man's behavior and thought processes. Some have dreamed and acted on theories which have isolated them into a cocoon-like existence safe from and blind to the realities of contemporary life. Others have woven tapestries of thought so thick as to prevent them from seeing ahead; they can only look backward. Others see ahead but not very clearly, for they carry with them irrelevant and burdensome remnants of the past. These are the more venturesome who are taxed for new answers, as are the few who even more thoroughly have abandoned traditional ways of thinking and treating patients. These are the few whose creativity is challenged to the utmost and who most need our support. Perhaps they are the current adolescents of psychiatry.

Some have retained their theories and ways so unaltered that they serve as a kind of security blanket. Their positions are unshakable as they account for every human phenomenon with an equanimity derived from an abiding faith, no matter what the social circumstances, struggles, and changes swirling about them. Accordingly, as has been so well described by Rinsley, they adhere to the *turmoil* view of adolescence.[3] According to them, adolescence is at best a period of psychological disturbance and "normative crisis." They describe the adolescent of our times as being in a state of identity crisis, or role diffusion, of storm and stress and ego exhaustion. They assume that all adolescents are somewhat disturbed or ill, in such a state of flux as to be undiagnosable, unanalyzable because they are unmotivated, and best permitted to reach adult years before a serious attempt is made to treat them in depth. These analysts view the subdued adolescent with suspicion because he is devoid of the symptoms he is supposed to have according to their theory of development.

The adolescent fits—or is fitted to—the theoretical framework which is supposed to account for his psychosexual and psychosocial development. If he abhors current social conditions, favors idealism and rejects the ways of authority figures, and particularly if he engages in violence, he is acting out and in rebellion against the castrating father figure. Were he aware of these seething forces within his unconscious, he would be more reasonable, for conduct of this nature has nothing to do with ideals, human values, or an appreciation of the dehumanizing aspects of the current scene. His behavior is considered less than rational and easily explicable, and, in effect, attenuated by classic psychoanalytic interpretation.

In recent years the views of the turmoil school have been seriously questioned by some psychiatrists as perhaps being pertinent only for the obviously disturbed, if not psychotic, adolescent, but certainly not applicable to the general adolescent population, which is regarded as being relatively stable and not alienated. These colleagues see adolescents at the extremes of the spectrum as being sick rather than in a state of "adjustment reaction" out of which they will grow in the ordinary course of events. They see such adolescents as diagnosable and in dire need of treatment for the schizophrenic process with which most of them suffer. In this regard, I believe with Rinsley, that the turmoil view of adolescence cannot be accepted as valid for the majority—if any—of the young. I agree with Masterson, that the adolescents showing serious pathology usually thought to be an "identity crisis" are in the main schizophrenic. They must be recognized and treated as such if they are to have a chance to recover, for they will not just "grow out of it."

If I read Rinsley[3] and Masterson[4] correctly, they have been developing new ideas and techniques, yet their basic beliefs seem rooted in unsupported theory. They tend to see the schizophrenic disorders of adolescence as fitting into one of two groups: (1) the "presymbiotic psychosis of adolescence," supposedly based on a failure of "normal" mother-infant symbiosis, which is believed to occur between the third and fifth months of life; and (2) the "symbiotic psychosis of adolescence," which is considered to be based on its continuation as such rather than on a "separation individuation." In other words, they say that if the normal mother-child symbiosis is not made, or if it is made and a "separation individuation" is not achieved, schizophrenia of one sort or another will occur in adolescence. This, too, I believe, is stretching to explain these phenomena within our accustomed theoretical framework. Facetiously, if I may, I would call it the "damned if you don't and damned if you do and then don't undo" theory. It is too pat. I cannot believe it really explains the origins of the psychopathology we see in adolescents, for it leaves too much uncovered and overlooked. I am not at all convinced by the evidence thus far that between the age of three and five months the infant forms a symbiotic relation with its mother, nor am I taken with the idea that any failure in separation individuation is a basic cause of adolescent psychopathology. There is much more involved, as an exploration of Arieti's recent ideas will show.[9] My conviction about the importance of interdependence to mental health forces me to question the value of conceptualizing in terms of separation individuation because of its overtones.

The Academy of Psychoanalysis was slowly and painfully planned over a period of years by those who broke from tradition for a variety of reasons. Among them was the thirst for academic freedom, the opportunity to be creative and innovative and to offer a serious forum for fresh ideas. One might say—and some did say—that the founders of the Academy had not been successfully analyzed, were rebellious and acting as adolescents in their undertaking. In fact, however, though they had some similar aims, they did have, and continue to have, widely different ideas about the origins and treatment of psychopathology.

I believe that there is no end to man's creativity and that what he carries in his cranium is the most delicate of organs. Our current theories to explain its psychodynamics are hardly sufficient to account for its complexities, powers, and potential. Its flexibility and ability to comprehend differently with new experience and knowledge is unending. It is the most rapidly changing of organs and is infinitely more complex and responsive than our most sophisticated computers. The external world—past, present, and unfolding, to which it is ceaselessly responding—is equally complicated, particularly the fellow human beings with whom one is constantly relating. While man takes on his nature as living matter from his environment—including that in utero— he derives his nature as a human being from others with whom he interacts. Thus he is entirely in debt to his fellow man for his existence as a "human." This is a difficult debt to appreciate and repay.

One of the keystones of psychoanalysis is the theory of the unconscious. As is true for some other theories, this one has been so universally accepted that we generally talk of it as a fact, not as a theory or a concept. We marvel at and speak of the "discovery" of the "unconscious," but the only thing factual about the unconscious is that it is taken as an unquestioned fact—though it is never seen, felt, measured, or even converted into a measurable form. It undeniably helps us to explain things, but too often it merely explains them away. Sometimes I imagine the field of psychoanalysis without the concept of the unconscious. I wonder and struggle to explain human phenomena in other terms and with other "theory." I strain to find and try techniques of treatment not influenced by any thoughts of the "unconscious." It is a difficult exercise, but I commend it to you as an effort worth trying, if only for a day. Sometimes I find it as difficult as I imagine it would be for a devoutly religious person to understand life without believing in God.

The challenge we face is to construct a theoretical model more appropriate to and consistent with the vast body of new knowledge and experience we have gathered and the innumerable new techniques we have successfully used. Despite these, we seem incapable of detaching ourselves from a theory born in another era and expressed by men of a different order of experience and knowledge. This compels us to fit the new into an old mold and hinders our creativity, so that our vision of human and social phenomena is not as clear as it might be. The practice of psychoanalysis today is so different from the original from which its theory grew that on this basis alone a new theoretical framework would seem in order. If we are innovative enough to so radically change our techniques and clinical practice, what is it that prevents us from altering our theoretical formulations? This inability may very well be responsible for our relative ineptness with serious psychopathology, as with that found in adolescents. This state of affairs obstructs our freedom to forge ahead.

Man has the capacity to incorporate his past in the acculturating process and to use his current state of awareness to see into the future. In the light of what he anticipates as a consequence of any behavior he contemplates, he judges what he will or will not do or may or may not do or what he dare or dare not do. It is his current awareness of reality and foresight which determine his behavior, rather than necessarily his past and "unconscious storehouse." If his awareness and judgment of past, present, and future are faulty and distorted, his decisions and actions will be accordingly inappropriate. Thomas has covered this view in his paper, "Purpose Versus Consequence in the Analysis of Behavior."[5] Psychiatrists assume that there is an underlying motive for every irrational act and that such behavior could not occur unless the patient possessed a purpose and aim, which is usually unconscious.

Freud stated that "The symptoms of neurosis are exclusively . . . either a substitutive satisfaction of some sexual impulse or measures to prevent such a satisfaction, and are, as a rule, compromises between the two—theoretically there is no objection to supposing that any sort of instinctual demand whatever could occasion these same repressions and their consequences."[6] Accordingly, he believed that all thought and behavior, normal and abnormal, were determined by underlying and unconscious purposes.

Psychodynamics has been described as "concerned with understanding the motives of human behavior."[7] Unfortunately, all schools of psychoanalytic thought to date, says Thomas, and I agree, maintain this chief concern. Levy also states: "The motivational viewpoint . . . has become ascendant. It is represented by a variety of patterns in the different schools of thought. Essentially, however the patterns may differ, the basic question is the same. What are the motives?"[8]

This may be said for the pioneers, from Alexander through Sullivan, Fromm-Reichman, and even Horney. In the main, not only was the emphasis on motivation, which had its roots in the unconscious and instinctual forces or the intrapsychic processes related to them, but the wellsprings were either in the past or in self-serving goals. Few left room for human values, elevated, ideal, and distinct from instinctual and underlying human passions. Since anatomy was destiny, conflict and struggle were inevitable and unalterably of a nature destructive to mankind and its strivings toward humaneness. Pessimism was the core of this approach. It is not difficult to see, then, the problems of applying it to the psychotherapy of the adolescent—filled with ideals, forward-looking, unbound by tradition or seeking freedom from its fetters, seething with passion for the suffering, and inclined to carry a flower rather than a gun toward his fellowman.

All of this is said to convey some of what we must have in mind when we consider inhospital treatment of the adolescent who is, in the main, schizophrenic. There are many critical factors which enter into his intensive psychotherapy. The values, attitudes, basic theoretical beliefs, and humaneness with which we approach the inpatient will be of the utmost importance. Our aims for him, as well as for ourselves, will be of equal importance. The technique of the psychotherapy will, of course, be critical but of hardly greater consequence than the milieu in which it is practiced. In other words, the two are inseparable and interpenetrating, so that one may hardly be considered apart from the other. The quality of "intensiveness" of the psychotherapy cannot be measured by the frequency of sessions or their duration in terms of minutes spent in a dyadic relationship. It may be quantified only by the intensity of the multitude and quality of the "human" relationships which exist in the hospital and by when and how they come to bear on the patient. A patient may be seen seven hours a week in a hospital setting without the therapy having an intensive quality in the sense I mean. However, the intensity and devotion with which the total professional team works together and approaches its task of treating the patient; the manner in which this team deals with and relates to the nonprofessional staff, who are also responsible for the patient's milieu; the quality of the value system which pervades the environment; the goals the professional staff has for the patient, for example, to merely render him symptom-free and return him quickly to society or establish a lengthy human relationship with him, intended to make him a more humanized individual better fit to survive the onslaughts of the society to which he must return; the ability of the team to arrive at and maintain a consensus about goals, and thereby milieu stability; the therapist's attitudes toward and involvement with the patient's family; and finally, the quality of the relationship between the therapeutic and administrative staffs, for example, the harmony and mutuality of purpose with which they work for the patient's welfare. All of these features are important to the intensive psychotherapy of the adolescent.

Beyond these factors, all of the human resources and forces must be highly organized and interrelated by a good communications network. They must be focused on the patient—who is really the only reason for the organization's existence. All must take into account the variety of groups present and the processes of their interaction. It is very important that patients *and* staff realize that they comprise a social structure, a society with a history, mores, laws, and values, a social system whose viability and success in achieving its goals depends on the ability of its members to relate to each other as humanly as possible. They must realize that as a group they have a goal before them, that of achieving a high degree of cohesiveness, which may always tantalize them by being in mind and in sight, but yet always beyond their grasp. Nonetheless, they must avoid the pessimism which could gnaw at and destroy them all. The task, of course, is made formidable by the difficulties the adolescent presents as an inpatient in intensive psychotherapy.

I return now to my earlier allusion to Arieti's work, but first a few preliminary remarks. I am sure that others, too, have noted that those among us who have gained our recognition for their prolonged, intensive, and effective work with schizophrenics have certain human qualities. They have developed through their work with these patients a great sensitivity to them and what they describe as their suffering. They develop deep feeling and loyalty to them and consider them to have capacities to see what the normal person overlooks. They observe fountains of creativity and find it rewarding to extend themselves limitlessly to salvage them. They do not despair, as most psychiatrists are prone to do with the schizophrenic and as did Freud who taught that they were not "fit subjects" for analysis, incapable of forming a transference relationship. It is these psychiatrists I am talking about who find new understanding of psychodynamics, develop new techniques of treatment, and venture forward and far afield in their quest to alleviate the schizophrenic's suffering.

In addition to inherent talents and unusual knowledge they gained from extensive work with the schizophrenic, these psychoanalysts built on the writings of pioneers who broke the bonds of tradition and learned from changing social conditions and values. The credit due them, however, is not diminished, and I know the reader is familiar with the names of those to whom I allude. For the purpose of this article, though, I would like to single out some of the ideas expressed by Arieti in a yet unpublished paper entitled "Psychotherapy of Schizophrenia."

Arieti believes that all psychiatrists, knowingly or unknowingly, are performing psychotherapy with schizophrenics, that the study of the interpersonal does not detract from the significance of the intrapsychic, that the schizophrenic's suffering is internal and that this sets up intrapsychic mechanisms which further alter interpersonal relations, and that as long as the human drama is interpersonal or social and not internalized in "abnormal" ways which injure the self, schizophrenia does not occur. Arieti has modified his former position and now believes that no more than 25 percent of mothers fit the image of the schizophrenogenic mother. He wonders why all psychiatrists believe patients' distorted portrayals of their mothers and discounts the possibility that they had "personal psychologic needs" to generalize what occurs only in a minority of cases. I think, as with Freud's need to believe the fantasies of his patients, and not to anyone's discredit, that it is conceivable that psychiatrists did and do have psychologic reasons for believing their patients' misconceptions. This is particularly true of that generation of psychiatrists who cling to the dyadic model and religiously refuse to see mothers and fathers personally to judge for themselves. We indicated this in 1958 in a paper on the subject of family therapy with the inpatient.[10] We saw too many normal parents of sick adolescents to accept the concept of the schizophrenogenic mother.

In returning to the basic question of why the patient distorts the parental image originally, Arieti resorts to this explanation: The mother does have some negative characteristics; the child becomes particularly sensitized to them because they are the ones that hurt; he ignores the others which are positive; and, making use of primary process cognition, the patient permits and perpetuates this partial awareness, or "part-object" relationship. Thus Arieti turns to traditional theory, which to my uneasy mind still leaves open to question the reason for the original distortion of reality—the inability to give precedence to the mother's positive attributes, and for that matter, those of people in general, particularly as the years elapse.

Arieti is in the forefront of those doing psychotherapy with the schizophrenias. He is original in his ideas for better understanding of them and creative in his techniques for their therapy. Many of these, which are derived from office practice, are applicable to the inpatient treatment of adolescents, most of whom are schizophrenic. First, Arieti says that other aspects of psychotherapy such as the manner of relating between the therapist and patient are more important than the psychodynamic understanding of the past and present. While others have thought similarly, Arieti refers here to "transference and countertransference interacting simultaneously." He believes that countertransference, contrary to classic theory, is not a complication to be avoided but "a necessary element in the treatment of the psychotic. Without intense feelings for the patient on the part of the therapist, no relatedness is established." This is a radical and laudatory departure from tradition, with which I am in complete agreement and which we have implemented for many years in the hospital treatment of our adolescent schizophrenics.

By far more innovative is another belief we share with Arieti, though our application is to the inpatient, while his is to the ambulatory. We have implemented it by building it into the hospital's social structure and living it with the patient. This idea is that the therapist, to quote Arieti, "share and combat" the patient's anxiety, and convey "the feeling that the burden" of the patient is also borne by the therapist. These beliefs are so contrary to those prevailing that I am sure they are not accepted by most psychoanalysts.

There is another area in which we agree with an uncommon belief held by Arieti. This is the belief that intensive psychotherapy requires the sharing of values which become common to both therapist and patient after arduous search and work. Initially their respective values are quite different, but apparently the successful process of psychotherapy requires their harmonization. Thus we have a system of values in the hospital, developed by all who have been engaged in it through the years, which we attempt to have the new patient share with us. Arieti holds this to be true for the office treatment of the psychotic, as well as "for any healthy human encounter." He believes, further, that the therapist must achieve a "peer" position with his patient and that this is possible only if they share values. I have some reservations about seeking a "peer relation" with patients, despite my agreement otherwise.

Apparently the schizophrenic has a singular sensitivity to the hostility rampant in society, which may very well play a part in producing his paranoid reactions. I agree with Arieti, however, that schizophrenia is an illness—an abnormal reaction to an abnormal situation—not a normal reaction to an unhealthy situation, as some tend to believe. Naturally, one's basic belief here will determine the nature of the inpatient program he establishes for the schizophrenic adolescent.

No one who works for a long period with the mentally ill is immune from developing a philosophy of treatment. Those who for years expose themselves to the schizophrenic often go beyond this to develop a "philosophy of life." They cannot escape a feeling relation to the schizophrenic because he suffers so, so they adopt even more than a parental role. They talk and feel in human-relationship terms and develop an enormous sympathy for the patient, who seems to evoke their most humane qualities. They tend to condemn the hostile world which renders the patient so helpless, seeing it as a jungle in which the schizophrenic cannot survive, although he is aware of its evil elements, particularly that of power. His anguished voice is a constant reminder of the inimical powers which prevail, and, says Arieti, "the therapist must hear this voice" which is actually calling for basic human values. Arieti says this power can be checked only by "human will," that we can help the patient only "if he experiences us as human beings who share his values and as peers." The patient's main goal is "not that of fighting persecutors, but of fighting evil and searching for love and fulfillment. Thus, his first and ultimate values will also be our values." This quote speaks for itself, as does Arieti's apparent faith in the "intangible universal values of individualism." The crucial point, however, is the human alliance evoked by the schizophrenic and sought openly by the therapist on behalf of the patient and, apparently, himself. The operating principle is the same for the inpatient adolescent; as a suffering schizophrenic he draws on the best in us.

I have much sympathy for this actively human approach, though a somewhat different philosophy of life, insofar as my main focus, with regard to values, is less individualistic. Naturally, we have conceptualized and implemented our inpatient program accordingly. The essence of it is in a paper entitled "Humanization and the Inpatient Therapeutic Process." (See Chapter 1.)

Our psychiatric hospital is regarded as a society in which professionals and patients relate to each other in various ways, including the dyadic psychotherapeutic, with an awareness that the nature of all these relationships will determine the course the patient's illness, if not his life, will take. Accordingly, how the one treats the other as a human being helps him understand and determine the direction the mental disorder takes within the confines of that society. We tend to think that certain social circumstances, as well as the schizophrenic process, have to some degree dehumanized the patient and that a hospital should accordingly supply counterbalancing humanizing influences. Consequently, those involved in the patient's treatment are emotionally tied to him; they are openly concerned about his welfare as a human being and utilize the hospital's value system to influence the patient's values in the direction of achieving some common ground for them. The hospital's values are part of its written law and mores, which the patient ultimately must share with us at least to some extent if he is to make progress as a human being, over and above symptomatic improvement. In this respect we agree with Arieti that the "relatedness" between patient and therapist is an aspect of psychotherapy more important than the psychodynamic understanding of past and present. We stress, however, that in hospital implementation there are a multitude of positive relationships. Many of them are psychotherapeutic, particularly if the social organization of the hospital is stable and has a value system which is consciously brought to bear as a "human" influence on the patient.

Our values call for not mere sensitivity to the hostility rampant in the world but sensitivity to the needs of fellow human beings, and beyond that, the motivation needed to satisfy those needs. This is not a value the adolescent schizophrenic can easily adopt. Our values often require the submergence of one's individual needs for those of the group. The human interaction and sacrifice of "individual liberty" which this often demands is most unsettling to the adolescent schizophrenic.

We equate functioning on an adult healthy level with stability, structured and productive activity. These are also aims that are difficult for the schizophrenic to come by and accept as associated with certain human values. We tend to take it for granted that, at least initially, we know better what the patient requires and act with patience, yet persistence and protectiveness, to do what we believe is in his best interest. We are ready to "interfere" with his "freedom" when that state might mean the "liberty" to injure himself or another, an act which might very well traumatize him forever. These attitudes we have, and actions we take in human relation to the patient we regard not merely as important ingredients of the psychotherapeutic process but as significant to the active humanizing process in which the adolescent schizophrenic needs engagement. The hospital's social system and pattern of treating with its inhabitants, including its patients, is part of the psychotherapeutic process. The patient's dyadic psychotherapeutic relationship is but one of a multitude of relationships in which he is engaged. All are directed toward the patient's development on a higher level as a human being—his humanization.

REFERENCES

1. Gralnick, A. "Psychotherapeutic and interpersonal aspects of insulin treatment." *Psychiatric Quarterly,* 18:179–96 (April 1944).
2. Schacht, L., and M. Blacker. "Leadership effect on the staff conference process." *Archives of General Psychiatry,* 20:358–64 (March 1969).
3. Rinsley, D. R. "A contribution to the nosology and dynamics of adolescent schizophrenia." *Psychiatric Quarterly,* 46:159–86 (1972).
4. Masterson, J. F. "Treatment of the adolescent with borderline syndrome: a problem in separation-individuation." *Bulletin of the Menninger Clinic,* 35:5–18 (1971).
5. Thomas, A. "Purpose versus consequence in the analysis of behavior." *American Journal of Psychotherapy,* 25:49–64 (January 1970).
6. Freud, S. *An outline of psychoanalysis.* New York: Norton, 1937, p. 85.
7. Report of 1952 Conference on Psychiatric Education. "The psychiatrist, his training and development." Washington, D.C.: American Psychiatric Association, 1953, p. 16.
8. Levy, D. "Capacity and motivation." *American Journal of Orthopsychiatry,* 27:1 (1957).
9. Arieti, S. "Psychotherapy of schizophrenia." Unpublished.
10. LeFebvre, P., J. Atkins, J. Duckman, and A. Gralnick. "The role of the relative in a psychotherapeutic program." *Canadian Psychiatric Association Journal,* 3:110–18 (1958).

PART THREE
CLINICAL RESEARCH

Chapter 14
Five-Hundred Case Study in a Private Psychiatric Hospital: Further Considerations in Evaluation

in collaboration with Rustu Yemez, M.D., Faruk Turker, M.D., Peter Schween, M.D., and Maurice Greenhill, M.D.

A degree of curiosity, mystery, and misconception generally characterizes the private (particularly the proprietary) psychiatric hospital despite our excellent means of communication and the rigorous standards of state and national accrediting bodies which these hospitals meet.

It occurred to the authors that there would be merit in holding a mirror to the face of such a hospital. The reflection might be enlightening to the many interested in the general field of hospital care for the mentally ill, as well as to the few of us involved in guiding the destinies of the scrutinized institution. Some want to "really know" what goes on behind the so-called walls of that private hospital set aside for "the rich"—"tucked away in the country" and so "inaccessible" to the professional and lay public.

More to the point, of course, are the following questions: What type of patient does it treat? How long does it treat him? How and why does it treat him so? What are the hospital's problems and their origins? Over which problems does the staff have control? When are they helpless and why? What are their handicaps? Which factors contribute to the patient's progress, which to his regression? What social forces are affecting these

169

hospitals, and toward what ultimate end? How do these forces then affect the sick they care for? Are there really differences between them and the public institutions? What are they? What are the differences among the private hospitals? What is the difference between a voluntary and a proprietary psychiatric hospital?

First, certain facts[1-6] about our hospital need to be known. At the time these 500 cases were in the hospital, the program was devoted to dynamically oriented psychotherapy in a "psychotherapeutic community atmosphere." It was supported by the wide use of drug therapy, family therapy, occupational and recreational therapy, and the incidental use of electroshock. Patients were rather carefully selected to exclude those under 16 or over 65, the organic and acutely addicted, and those seeking "two or three weeks of hospitalization." Instead, the program sought the patient and family who realized that more than two or three weeks were needed for an effective result and wanted greater stability for the patient and change in the family situation. The emphasis was on basic change for the better rather than on symptom alleviation and the quickest return to the community. Each of the average census of 40 patients received at least three hours per week of individual psychotherapy. A team of seven full-time therapists acted as a "closed staff" fully responsible for the total program and was supported by approximately 60 people in the other departments.

This study really set out to do an ongoing evaluation of the clinical work of High Point Hospital. Inherent in this endeavor was the intention to develop procedures whereby evaluation could become standardized and continuous. This meant that we had to be prepared for change, for modification in record-keeping, for reorganizing clinical procedures, for the possible discovery and exposure of error, clinical bias, and employment of value judgment, and ready with the courage to acknowledge this to ourselves.

Demographic studies of a statistical nature occur in number in the literature related to public and voluntary private hospitals.[7-10] We know of no such report in depth in connection with a proprietary hospital. Yet such material would appear to have value to the mental health field as a whole, not only from the standpoint of clinical psychiatry, but also of community organization and planning in mental health. This would seem particularly true in light of the Federal Medicare program and associated state programs which expand the segment of the population treated under them.

It was our intention to canvass all possible categories of data in our demographic studies, starting with the most obvious (patent) and proceeding to the most subtle (hidden) which might be influential in determining hospital procedures and results. Our goal was more a pursuit of results in terms of the processing of data according to clinical, administrative, sociological, and interpersonal categories, plus an assessment of their interrelationships. This report, then, deals with the more obvious (patent) variables, both for their own value and for their assistance in leading us to the more hidden variables, so that these, in turn, may later be studied with truer relevancy.

PROCEDURE

In early 1961 preliminary conferencing by the research staff decided (1) that the first five years of the hospital's existence should be regarded as its period of stabilization, and that the records of its second five-year period would be studied, (2) that a prepared and determined list of data (variables) would be culled from these records, (3) that one member of the research team would study most of the records and oversee the work of others who might also gather data, and (4) that as the data were gathered regular conferences by the research team would be held to direct and develop the study.

During the first two years an average of two hours was spent on each of the hospital records of the 500 patients admitted in the six-year period starting in 1956. Data from these records were collected on prepared individual forms which covered all possible categories dealing with patent variables. These were selected by research-group consensus and continually tested out. Some 30 exploratory tables, graphs, and correlations were developed. These, together with the individual forms, were considered the raw data.

The third year was spent in refining and revalidating the raw data. Omissions, lack of differentiation, or weak definition of clinical fact in a few records led to modifying or eliminating some categories to insure validity. Each investigator's collection of data was checked by one and sometimes two other workers; where there was lack of agreement, final decision was reserved for consensual validation by the research team. A paper was written during this time to collate and record our preliminary thinking and the research methodology involved in preparation for this particular report.[11]

All of this finally led to the creation of a new research-data form to guide the refining of the data and to be used in the ongoing evaluation of each subsequent patient's record. The data on these forms were grouped into four major classifications: (1) Identifying data, (2) Illness, (3) Course of present hospitalization, and (4) Outcome. The data under these classifications were evaluated by the research group as a whole under the following headings:

    (a) assessment of total figures
    (b) assessment of trend over the years considered
    (c) significant change at any point
    (d) comparison with other studies
    (e) consideration of the possible reasons for the results in (a) through (d).

I. Identifying of Background Social Data

Constant factors which could be checked with validity were sex, age, residence, marital status, religion, education, and occupation. These were collated in their own right and later cross-checked or correlated with treatment variables included in this study.

A. Sex vs. Number and Percentage of Patients by Years
From 1956 to 1961 the ratio of female to male patients was two to one (66.2 percent female and 33.8 percent male). There was no changing trend during these years.

The average population of private and voluntary hospitals in

New York State shows a similar ratio.[12] In the state's public hospitals the ratio of the sexes is one to one on first admission.[13] The reasons for this may lie in the fact that there seems to be a direct relationship between the hospitalization of females and high income, and conversely, a higher hospital rate for males where income is much lower.

B. Residence

Ninety percent of the patients came from the northeast. The trend remained fairly constant through the years. There are no significant trends in the patients coming from other areas of the country, except for the fact that there are fewer patients coming from the southeast during the last three years of the study than during the first three years, although this is not particularly significant. As for a breakdown of patients from the northeast, which is the major category, there seems to be a decrease of patients coming from New York City, with an associated increase in patients from Westchester County and other areas of the northeast. It is suggested that High Point is becoming more of a community hospital for Westchester County and/or the New York-New Jersey-Connecticut area.

C. Age

Fifty-two percent of the patients ranged in age from 20 to 40, and 72 percent were between 20 and 50, with the largest percentage (29.2) in the 30–39 bracket. Perhaps the most striking feature of trend by age was the increase in the adolescent population after 1958. During the six-year period the following movement in adolescent population was noted (in percent): 1956—7, 1957—5.4, 1958—4.8, 1959—13.5, 1960—12, and 1961—11, with an overall 9 percent adolescents in the 500 cases studied. The average was 18.8 percent for patients 50 and over.

D. Marital Status

The marital status of the 500 patients studied was (in percent):

Single	Married	Widowed	Separated	Divorced
29.6	57.2	3.6	3.2	6.4

E. Religion

The population was predominantly Jewish, as shown in Table 1.

Table 1. Religion—Percentage of Patients by Years

Religion	1956	1957	1958	1959	1960	1961	Average
Protestant	18.8	21.5	16.9	20.0	22.4	29.2	21.2
Catholic	17.8	17.7	15.7	11.4	12.0	14.6	15.0
Jewish	59.4	58.3	67.4	54.5	59.6	51.3	59.4
Others	4.0	2.5	.0	9.1	6.0	4.9	4.4

The percentage of Jewish patients was in the area of 60 percent, with a peak of 67.4 percent in 1958 and a decline to 51.3 percent in 1961. In the peak year two-thirds were Jewish (67.4 percent) and one-third Christian (32.6 percent). In 1961, the ratios approached 1:1, with 51.3 percent Jewish and 43.8 percent Christian. This did not indicate a trend toward the admission of more Christian patients any more than the 1958 figures denoted a trend toward an increase in the rate of admission of Jewish patients.

The higher incidence of Jewish patients may be due to the proximity of the hospital to New York City, with its large Jewish population, although other psychiatric hospitals in the New York area have patients predominantly of other faiths. One might speculate whether this finding had to do with the religion of the hospital's medical director, although the clinical directors and resident staff were non-Jewish in those years. At any rate, religion is a variable which might have to be taken into account in assessing hospital milieu and results.

F. Education

The patient population, on the whole, was a highly educated group—58.4 percent had college education (complete and incomplete) and 33.6 percent were college graduates.

The trend was for the sum of the high school graduate patients to drop over the years, whereas the number of college-educated increased. This would reflect the fact that all psychiatric hospitals are admitting increasing numbers of young adults.

Table 2. Education—Percentage of Patients by Years

Education	1956	1957	1958	1959	1960	1961	Average
Under 12 grades	12.8	14.0	21.7	16.0	16.4	14.6	15.8
High school graduate	32.7	33.0	18.0	21.6	15.0	17.0	23.4
Over 12 grades	18.9	25.3	23.0	23.9	25.3	34.2	24.8
College graduate	34.6	22.7	33.7	35.2	41.8	34.2	33.6
Unascertained	1.0	5.0	3.6	3.3	1.5	0	2.4
Total	100	100	100	100	100	100	100

G. Occupation

The principal groups in the patient population, by occupation, were (1) housewives, (2) business and clerical workers, and (3) students, in that order. This is shown in the following table:

Table 3. Occupation—Percentage of Total Patients

Housewife	Business	Student	Professional	Labor	Artist	None	Total
43.4	19.4	17.0	8.8	4.4	1.4	7.6	100.0

Noteworthy was an increase in percentage of the student group over the years 1956–61, with a gradual increase from 8.92 percent in 1956 to 21.92 percent in 1961. This probably follows the increase in the percentage of adolescents over those years. The average number of physicians treated was in the neighborhood of 2–3 percent of the hospital population in any one year, with the exception of 1961, when it was 9.75 percent.

Demographic Profile of the High Point Hospital Patient

The typical patient is apt to be a young Jewish housewife from the northeast with a partial or complete college education. In recent years the patient is more likely than heretofore to be an adolescent of either sex and a college student. But the spectrum of patients is broad, embracing the major religious backgrounds and coming from a business or professional family.

II. Illness

A. Previous Psychotherapy

Over 70 percent of the patients had previous psychotherapy. The index for psychotherapy was taken to be any patient who had been involved in regularly scheduled sessions with a psychotherapist for three months or more. Table 4 indicates the distribution of previously treated cases.

Table 4. Previous Psychotherapy—Percentage of Patients

	1956	1957	1958	1959	1960	1961	Average
Previous psychotherapy	63.36	60.96	56.62	73.86	82.08	87.82	71.60
No psychotherapy	20.97	10.12	16.97	15.90	11.94	12.18	15.00
Unknown	15.83	20.25	25.30	10.27	5.96	0	13.40
Total	100	100	100	100	100	100	100

It is noteworthy that a large number of patients had records in which no notation had been made regarding this factor. This number was far greater during the first three years of the study than during the last three. In 1961 there were no "unknowns." We take this to reflect the improvement in record-keeping, especially after the study began in 1961. In that year, with a more careful recording system, 87.82 percent of the patients were noted to have been in psychotherapy at some time prior to their hospitalization. This suggests that we were dealing mainly with chronically troubled patients rather than those with recent disorders.

B. Number of Previous Hospitalizations

About half of the patients admitted in the period studied had not been hospitalized before, approximately one-fourth had been hospitalized only once previously, and 13.4 percent twice previously. Another 10 percent had been hospitalized three or more times. We might categorize this latter group as having a tendency toward chronic hospitalization. The trend over the years, in all of the categories, does not seem to be significant, and a table is therefore not shown.

It is interesting to note that many patients are hospitalized despite having had or being in the midst of psychotherapy. We may ask, at what point and with what considerations in mind patients are hospitalized. We hope to study this at a future date, as well as the correlation of previous psychotherapy and previous hospitalization with outcome of care at our hospital.

C. Diagnoses

Table 5 shows that the largest category of diagnosis is schizophrenia, approximately 68 percent of the patients in the five

Table 5. Diagnosis—Percentage of Patients by Years

	1956	1957	1958	1959	1960	1961	Average
Schizophrenia	68.01	72.2	63.9	68.2	71.6	61.0	67.8
Psychoneuroses	13.9	7.6	9.0	15.9	10.5	17.0	12.6
Affective disorders	7.9	5.6	8.4	4.6	3.0	6.0	6.0
Personality disorders	4.0	3.9	9.0	2.3	6.0	8.5	5.6
Involutional psychosis	3.0	7.6	8.4	6.8	3.0	4.8	5.4
Other psychoses	3.2	3.1	1.3	2.2	5.9	2.7	2.6

years having this disorder. The category next in frequency is psychoneuroses, with 12.6 percent. Personality disorders, affective disorders, and involutional psychosis each have approximately 5–6 percent. Almost 80 percent of the patients were diagnosed as having psychotic reactions (schizophrenia, affective disorders, involutional psychosis).

There is some indication that as the percentage of depressive reactions went up in a given year, the percentage of schizophrenia went down, as if there were an inverse relationship. In 1958 and 1961 there was a considerable drop in the schizophrenic category. The recollection of the research group is that in those years some of the staff physicians found it more difficult generally to make a diagnosis of schizophrenia because of differences in their concept of that disorder. Diagnoses were made by the individual patient's therapist with the signed concurrence of the medical director.

A comparison with other statistics indicates that we make the diagnosis of schizophrenia much more often than other psychiatric hospitals. Licensed hospitals in the State of New York reported approximately 30 percent of their populations as being schizophrenics.[14] For the United States as a whole (1960) about 22 percent of the patients in private hospitals were diagnosed as schizophrenia and/or paranoid reactions[15]—less than one-third of those so diagnosed at High Point Hospital.

These findings suggest several possibilities. High Point attracts more schizophrenic patients or its admission policies make for the selection of a greater number of such patients or the concept of what constitutes schizophrenia may differ from that of other institutions. On the other hand, it is just as likely that we are less apprehensive about making the diagnosis of schizophrenia because of greater optimism about its alleviation. Nevertheless, the findings will compel us to take an even closer look at our demographic, admission, and diagnostic practices in the future.

III. Course in Hospital

A. Type of Admission

The principal type of admission through the six-year period was by voluntary commitment (90 percent), followed by physician certifications (7 percent) and court certifications (2 percent). This proportion remained relatively constant until 1961, when voluntary admissions dropped to 80 percent and physician certifications rose to 18 percent. These figures approximate those for voluntary admission to licensed hospitals in the State of New York (85 percent).[16]

B. Chemotherapy

There was a decline in the use of tranquilizers through the six-year period. In general, close to three quarters of the patients were on tranquilizers during some part of their stay at the hospital. Throughout the period practically no antidepressants were used (the antidepressants came in as a new drug in 1957). The combined use of tranquilizers plus antidepressants increased markedly in the second three-year period.

The category "No medication" comprised 13.8 percent of

Table 6. Medication—Percentage of Patients by Years

	1956	1957	1958	1959	1960	1961	Avg.
Tranquilizers	81.2	70.0	84.3	57.5	67.2	58.6	72.2
Antidepressants	0	0	0	1.2	0	1.2	0.4
Tranquilizers and anti- depressants	0	8.8	3.6	33.1	23.9	15.8	13.6
No medication	18.9	21.5	12.0	8.0	9.9	12.2	13.8

the patients who were treated by psychotherapy and the therapeutic milieu alone. (A considerably higher percentage of
patients were treated without medication in 1956 and 1957.) The
13.8 percentage represents an "N" of 69 patients who had
psychotherapy alone, a reasonable sample to study in trying to
assess the results of psychotherapy. This at least points the way
for more careful consideration of such an assessment in our
future evaluations.

C. Electroconvulsive Therapy
The use of electroconvulsive therapy dropped steadily
throughout the six-year period, especially during the last three
years. In the six-year period, 13.2 percent of all patients
received E.C.T., ranging from 21 percent in 1956 down to 3
percent in 1959, 1960, and 1961. In more recent years this
percentage is even lower. Of those who had this type of therapy,
62 percent received fewer than 10 treatments.

D. Discharges
The majority of patients left "without medical approval."
Over the six years 55 percent of the patients did this, compared
to 34 percent who left with medical approval and 10 percent who
were transferred to other hospitals. The percentage transferred
to other hospitals seems high, but we have no figures from other
private psychiatric hospitals with which to compare this. It is
also noted that some patients leave against medical advice and
appear shortly thereafter in other hospitals. These might be
considered unofficial transfers which would actually raise the
transfer statistics if it were possible to obtain valid data on all
such "transfers." Reasons for official transfer with medical

Table 7. Type of Discharge—Percentage of Patients by Years

	1956	1957	1958	1959	1960	1961	Avg.
With medical approval	42.5	35.4	30.1	40.9	32.8	19.5	34.0
Without medical approval	49.5	43.0	60.2	48.9	61.2	70.7	55.2
Transferred	7.0	20.3	9.7	10.2	6.0	9.8	10.4
Other	1.0	1.3	0	0	0	0	0.4

approval included change to a state hospital, change to custodial hospitals in the case of "hopeless" patients, transfer to lower-cost institutions, and movement of patients closer to home.

Discharge Without Medical Approval

Since this was a striking factor, it was assessed more closely. The trend of such discharge climbed sharply from 1957 on (43 to 70 percent). In 1956, 42.5 percent left with medical advice, and by 1961 only 19.5 percent did so. In 1961, 70.7 percent left without medical concurrence.

In order to understand the reason for this, the source of responsibility for patients leaving in this manner was examined.

Other authors have studied the matter of discharges against medical advice.[17-19] Most of such discharges in our hospital were the result of patient pressure to leave prematurely, approximately 33 percent of patients leaving that way in comparison to 20 percent responding to family pressure, and 12.6 percent influenced by financial pressure. The tendency for patient pressure to operate against our advice to stay for further improvement remained constant until 1961, when it increased markedly.

Table 8. Source of Discharge as Percentage of Total Yearly Discharges

	1956	1957	1958	1959	1960	1961	Avg.
Patient's pressure	26.7	25.3	35.0	33.0	28.3	48.8	32.8
Family pressure	18.8	17.7	15.7	15.9	25.4	29.3	20.2
Financial pressure	12.9	38.0	19.3	6.8	13.4	19.5	12.6
Referring doctor's pressure	1.0	0	0	0	0	0	0.2
Unknown source	40.6	19.0	30.0	44.3	32.9	2.4	34.2

Family pressure for premature discharge also remained fairly constant until 1961, when it also increased. It is noted, however, that in 1961 the unknown sources of discharge against advice dropped markedly to a low of 2.4 percent. Either the nature of patient and family pressure was more obvious in that year or the staff had become aware of the problem and were more skillful in assessing and recording it, if not in combating it. We suspect it is for the latter reason.

Resistance to insight therapy is a well-known fact. In a hospital setting it will be masked in various ways. The patient will use his improvement to insist that he is well enough to leave, especially since he has "other obligations, too"; the family, especially if engaged in family therapy with the patient, will find its own rationalizations, particularly financial ones, to press its point that the patient is "ready enough to leave," albeit prematurely. However, when a medical staff is devoted to thorough therapy and seeks meaningful reconstruction rather than superficial compensation, it must withhold its approval. In most instances it does so even if the patient is visibly (though superficially) improved. In so doing it indicates the need for continued care of the patient.

IV. Outcome

A. Duration of Present Hospitalization
Sixteen percent of the patients stayed less than one month, the group demonstrating a consistent upward trend over the six years, from 4 to 22 percent.

It is surprising that a hospital which seeks "long-term"

Table 9. Duration of Stay—Percentage of Patients

	1956	1957	1958	1959	1960	1961	Avg.
Less than 1 month	4.0	13.9	18.1	20.5	20.9	22.0	16.0
1–3 months	36.6	34.2	33.8	22.7	29.9	25.6	30.5
3–6 months	36.6	27.8	25.3	22.7	20.9	31.9	28.0
6–12 months	6.9	11.3	17.0	19.3	23.9	14.4	17.2
12–24 months	5.8	5.6	4.8	9.1	4.5	6.1	6.2
Over 24 months	3.0	5.1	1.2	3.2	0	0	2.1

patients should have an average of 16 percent of them stay less than one month—an unsatisfactory situation. A host of factors, however, can account for this, the most prominent being error and miscalculation in the selection of the patient. Other factors have to do with patients eloping or becoming too disturbed for the general patient population or a family member becoming too distraught at the rupture of a symbiotic relationship. At times the hospital has merely been "used" by the family to control a bad situation at home or until the "more favored" hospital can admit the patient. Sometimes an unanticipated medical or surgical complication removes the patient rapidly. At any rate, this finding highlights the importance of patient selection in the fulfillment of the hospital's treatment goals. It taught us to improve our admission techniques so that in more recent years the percentage of patients who leave so quickly has dropped considerably.

About 30 percent of the patients stay one to three months, and an almost equal percentage (28) remain from three to six months. Only 8.2 percent stay over one year, and only 2 percent of those over two years. Approximately 45 percent of the patients stay between three and 12 months. The trends show an increase in the 6–12 months category in the last three years of the period studied.

Our devotion to intensive psychotherapy, applied long enough to achieve not mere remission but significant change, coupled with the fact that so many patients stay only one to three months (we here exclude from consideration those who stay less than one month), illustrates the gap between one's stated goal and his opportunity to fulfill it. These particular statistics give the hospital some of the quality of a brief treatment center. On the other hand, almost half the patients stay from three to 12 months or longer. These figures show that a range from brief to protracted therapy may take place, but, further, that in the private hospital one often has the fullest opportunity to fulfill his stated goal for patients.

B. Readmissions

The readmission rate stayed relatively constant through the first four years studied, at about 10 percent, but dropped to 7.5

percent in 1960 and 2.4 percent in 1961. The data could not help us explain these figures.

C. *Patient Grouping upon Discharge*

In our particular psychotherapeutic community, four patient groupings exist. These are structured as Groups I through IV, the patients of which are in differing states of convalescence, defined by clinical standards. In the succeeding groups to which he is assigned, each patient is given increased responsibility as his improvement occurs. Group I is comprised of the patients who are most ill, Group IV those who are most well.

Over the six-year period, more departing patients were from Group III than any other group. Over these same years the trend has been for the patients discharged from Group IV to drop from 62 percent in 1956 to 17 percent in 1961. The increasing percentage of patients discharged from Group III—and even Group II— is, of course, far from the ideal of discharging all patients from Group IV. The latter group is our most advanced—the one to which patients aspire for major "privilege and responsibility" in the patient-participation program, and one in which they can consolidate their gains. These facts would again illustrate that many patients have left prematurely, and without getting the full advantage of what the treatment program has to offer them. This fact, if general throughout hospitals, may help account for the relatively high relapse rate among psychiatric patients. It may be that we have here an excellent example of penny-wise, pound-foolish!

D. *Condition on Discharge*

Careful consideration has been given to the patient's condition on discharge according to criteria established by consensual validation on the part of the staff.

The figures would suggest that we tend to be conservative regarding the use of the term "much improved." The majority of patients (57.3 percent) fall in the "moderately improved" category, whereas only 13.2 percent were described as much improved. There seem to be no really significant trends through the years, other than that earlier there was a tendency to weight the condition on discharge more at the upper end of the "much

Table 10. Condition on Discharge—Percentage of Patients

	1956	1957	1958	1959	1960	1961	Avg.
Much improved	17.8	12.7	8.4	10.2	17.9	12.2	13.2
Moderately improved	69.3	49.4	62.6	59.1	58.2	45.1	57.3
Slightly improved	7.9	13.9	14.5	14.8	11.9	22.0	14.2
Unimproved	5.0	24.1	14.5	15.9	11.9	20.7	15.3

improved" and "moderately improved" scale, whereas in 1961 the weighting was in the direction of "slightly improved" and "unimproved." This could be due to the general level of illness of the group of patients in the hospital in the earlier and latter part of the six-year period, or due to the personal criteria by which the respective staffs of those times evaluated the patients.

A comparison of these findings with those of licensed private hospitals in the State of New York shows that these hospitals had an additional category termed "recovered."[20] It appears that either we do not achieve as good results or we are more conservative than others. In addition to not classifying schizophrenics as "recovered," we had a 13.2 percent "much improved" rate as compared to one of 30.5 percent in other hospitals. However, we do recognize that the "human factor" makes for wide variation in the evaluation of a patient's condition.

E. The Duration of Hospitalization vs. Length of Illness

The length of time a patient remains in the hospital will be determined by many factors besides the actual success of the form of treatment employed and the degree of the patient's improvement. Rarely is a patient as well as we might like him to be before circumstances dictate his discharge. This holds true in public as well as voluntary and proprietary hospitals. Some of these circumstances have already been suggested. Though economic factors are prominent, they are not always primary. The pressure for bed space, for instance, will weigh heavily in determining exactly when a patient is discharged. The "need" for the patient at home as determined by an emotionally torn relative is another factor. The patient's many resistances, particularly to insight therapy, also drive him to forego a full measure of hospital care. Many similar factors could be mentioned, including the nature and ability of the patient's psychiatrist.

The current theory in psychiatry that short-term treatment is best suggests to the patient that the less time he stays in the hospital, the better off he is and the less sick he is. Many now think that hospitalization, particularly if extended, makes the patient sicker. The emphasis on community psychiatry operates in the same direction. Sometimes one feels that there is something of a sense of competition among hospitals to see who can get patients out in the shortest average time. How stable the patient's improvement really is and how likely he is to remain out, let alone improve further, often seem to be less a matter for consideration. The ideal, of course, is for a patient to stay until a hospital program and its selected treatment forms achieve their maximum benefit and make possible the maximum prognosis that the patient will prosper in the environment to which he returns.

It is difficult to assess accurately the efficacy of any form of treatment or hospital program because there are so many variables other than duration of hospitalization. It is no wonder that confusion exists and that we tend to simplify things for ourselves by directly correlating the success of a specific form of treatment with the duration of hospitalization. The unfortunate part is the resulting tendency to equate brevity of hospitalization with "successful" outcome, even in the absence of good evaluative and follow-up studies. It is difficult to avoid the dilemma. The authors' particular problem in this area is compounded because we think of our "total program" (with its many treatment facets) as the therapeutic agent.

A study of statistics dealing with any form of treatment in psychiatry reveals a striking correlation between its success and the period of time a patient has been sick prior to the institution of therapy.[22-24] Awareness and study of why this is so may ultimately furnish understanding of the nature of mental illness, particularly schizophrenia and its treatment. It seems that this one factor, namely the duration of the illness (as well as the number of the attack in cases of schizophrenia), has most to do with the success of the treatment, in terms of the duration of hospitalization. With this in mind we thought we should see whether our study would reveal a similar correlation between the duration of illness and length of time our patients stayed in the hospital. We could then judge, or at least speculate whether our "total treatment program" operated as therapeutically as any of the more specific treatment forms.

The statistics presented in this article were refined and validated. We do want to point out that those presented in this particular section did not lend themselves to a similar validation and are therefore not as reliable. However, they would seem of some significance since they indicate trends in support of the general finding that the results (in terms of duration of hospitalization) of most forms of therapy are correlated with the length of the illness prior to treatment. The data presented in this section could not be validated for two main reasons. First, it is difficult to determine the exact onset of illness, particularly of schizophrenia. The matter is one that is often in dispute. Additionally, when more than one attack is involved, it is equally difficult to tell whether episodes are distinct or whether the second is really the continuation of the first with a period of quiescence rather than remission in between. Second, duration of hospitalization is so often determined by factors beyond the doctor's control rather than by his decision, that we believed this factor could not be validated by our retrospective study.

However, despite these considerations, we believed that in so large a study, the factors involved might more or less average out. The data could then have some significance, if only to indicate a trend. As it turns out, the findings show that a total treatment program (which emphasizes psychotherapy in combination with other treatment modalities in its psychotherapeutic community program) also shows the same result trends as more specific forms of treatment. Again, they suggest that the length of illness is decidedly related to the results (measured by duration of hospitalization), as is true with the specific modalities such as insulin and electroshock.

The following five tables emphasize two relationships: (1) the length of illness to the duration of hospitalization, and (2) the length of illness to the condition on discharge. These relationships are shown for the different numbers of episodes the patients had. It is evident for each category, with minor exception, that the longer a patient has been ill at the time of admission, the longer he remains in the hospital. This seems to be true, again with minor exception, regardless of the number of the attack. The statistics further show (for the first, second, and equivocal second or third attack categories) that the duration of hospitalization varies little when the length of illness is 0 to 6 months and 6 to 12 months. The variation definitely begins to show up in the 6-to-12 month length-of-illness category of the third episode. Here the duration of hospitalization goes up steeply. It is obvious that when the length of illness is more than one year, especially with the second and third episodes, the duration of hospitalization goes up most markedly. This is as we would expect and is analogous to the findings with insulin and electroshock therapy, namely, that when the patient is sick longer, he responds less readily to insulin and electroshock. The difference, of course, is that with these physiologic treatments, the patient sick too long does not respond no matter how long he is treated, *whereas these patients do seem to respond successfully with longer treatment in a program such as ours.*

The great majority of psychiatrists today have gained their basic knowledge of prognosis and results from two sources: (1) their clinical experience in state and federal institutions, and (2) the prevalent source of statistical studies, namely the public institutions. We have concluded from them that the longer a patient is ill, the worse is his prognosis and that the more episodes he has, the worse his chances of improving are. *Our own statistics, however, strongly suggest that we may now have reason to question such conclusions.*

Even a cursory look at Tables 11 to 14 will show that the level of improvement (percent moderately and much improved) of those ill for the longer periods of time is practically equal to that for those ill the shorter periods of time. And most surprising of all, this seems to hold true even for those in their second and third attacks.

Table 15, which includes all of the cases, shows that the percent of moderately to much improved patients remains about the same regardless of length of illness. However, the duration

Table 11. First Episode

Length of Illness (months)	No. of Cases	Duration of Stay (months)	% Unimproved & Slightly Imp.	% Moderately & Much Imp.
0–6	62	3.93	28.9	71.1
6–12	52	3.82	23.2	76.8
12–24	47	4.83	34.1	65.9
Over 24	51	5.49	31.4	68.6
Unascertained	8	2.76	50.0	50.0
Total	220	4.43	30.0	70.0

Table 12. Second Episode

Length of Illness (months)	No. of Cases	Duration of Stay (months)	% Unimproved & Slightly Imp.	% Moderately & Much Imp.
0–6	45	3.80	37.8	62.2
6–12	20	3.80	30.0	70.0
12–24	29	5.61	20.7	79.3
Over 24	13	7.37	38.5	61.5
Unascertained	1	18.60	100.0	0
Total	108	4.85	32.4	67.6

Table 13. Third Episode

Length of Illness (months)	No. of Cases	Duration of Stay (months)	% Unimproved & Slightly Imp.	% Moderately & Much Imp.
0–6	38	4.15	7.9	92.1
6–12	29	7.80	34.5	65.5
12–24	26	6.72	30.8	69.2
Over 24	17	11.70	35.3	64.7
Unascertained	4	6.65	25.0	75.0
Total	114	6.97	24.5	75.5

Table 14. Equivocal Second or Third Episode

Length of Illness (months)	No. of Cases	Duration of Stay (months)	% Unimproved & Slightly Imp.	% Moderately & Much Imp.
0–6	17	3.29	23.6	76.4
6–12	10	4.66	40.0	60.0
12–24	6	11.50	0	100.0
Over 24	22	3.29	13.6	86.4
Unascertained	1	2.30	100.0	0
Total	56	4.39	21.5	78.5

Table 15. Grand Totals

Length of Illness (months)	No. of Cases	Duration of Stay (months)	% Unimproved & Slightly Imp.	% Moderately & Much Imp.
0–6	162	3.88	25.9	74.1
6–12	111	4.93	28.8	71.2
12–24	108	5.86	27.8	72.2
Over 24	104	6.12	29.8	70.2
Unascertained	15	4.97	50.0	50.0
Total	500	5.11	28.5	71.5

of hospitalization required for them increases as their length of illness prior to treatment increases. What we surmise, of course, is that to achieve these better results an active treatment program must be pursued in the hospital for a longer period of time. We may at least say that longer periods of hospitalization are beneficial, not necessarily injurious. What may be true in the public, or custodial, type of institution is not true for the active, treatment hospital. In other words, and contrary to what we have believed, patients who have been ill longer and more frequently may have a prognosis equal to those who have been sick for shorter periods and less frequently. This is the reverse of general experience with insulin and electroshock therapy, namely, that the longer and more frequently a patient has been sick, the worse his prognosis with such treatment. The findings of this study, therefore, seem important, if only as a contrast to those we generally see emanating from the public institutions and upon which we have depended.

Figure 1 reflects Table 15 and shows that as the length of illness increases (in months), the duration of hospital treatment necessarily also increases. It covers all of the patients regardless of number of episode. Each "bar" shows the number of cases in each category (that is, 0 to 6 months, 6 to 12 months, etc.), and the height of the bar shows the duration of hospitalization in months. The dotted line indicates the average number of months of hospital treatment for all the patients.

Figure 2 breaks down the first four bars of Figure 1 into differently shaded subbars which indicate the number of the episode, that is, whether first, second, second or third, or third.

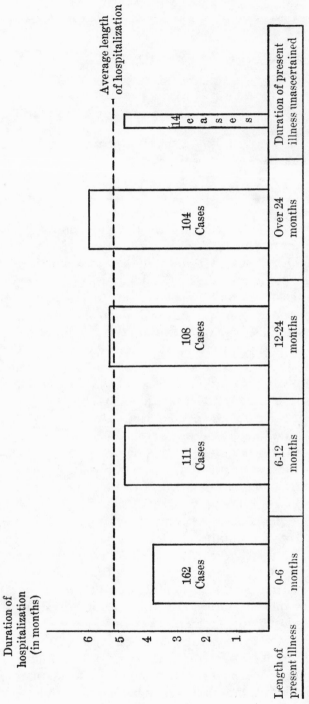

Figure 1. Overall Average Duration of Hospitalization vs. length of Illness (regardless of number of episodes)

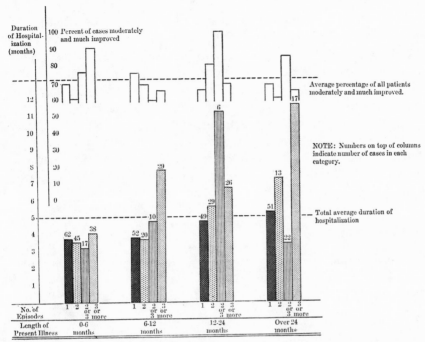

Figure 2. Length of Present Illness vs. Average Duration of Hospitalization and Percentage of Case With Moderate or Much Improvement

For instance, the first vertical-lined subbar shows 62 patients to have been in their first episode, and ill 0 to 6 months before hospitalization. These patients were hospitalized just short of four months. The second vertical-lined subbar shows 52 patients to have been in their first episode and ill 6 to 12 months before being hospitalized. These particular patients were also hospitalized just short of four months. The clear bars in the upper part of the graph indicate the percentage of cases "moderately to much improved." Thus, of the 62 patients in their first episode who were sick 0 to 6 months before hospitalization, 71 percent were "moderately to much improved." This is tabulated in Table 11. This interpretation of the graph may be followed throughout for each differently shaded subbar from left to right and for each clear bar above which refers to it. The essential point is that as the length of illness increases with each category of episode, the duration of hospital treatment also increases. With a treatment program such as is described here, however, the percentage of cases that do well stays equally high rather than diminishing as is usually shown in the statistics of public institutions for similar patients. The needed ingredient to accomplish these better results is probably the longer period of *such* hospital treatment. This may be seen by relating the respective subbars to the lower broken line which indicates in months the average duration of hospital treatment for all the patients.

Correlations

Certain factors were weighed against others to establish correlations which would allow a closer evaluation of some of the pertinent data. Of the correlations studied, the following appear to be most relevant:

(a) Duration of present hospitalization versus condition on discharge
(b) Type of discharge versus condition on discharge
(c) Diagnosis versus type of discharge.

(a) Duration of Present Hospitalization vs. Condition on Discharge

Seventy-eight patients (15.6 percent of the 500) stayed less than one month. Fully two-thirds of these left without medical consent and were described as "slightly improved" and "unimproved," and only one-third as "much" and "moderately improved." However, of the 154 patients (30.8 percent of the 500) who stayed 1 to 3 months, better than two-thirds (22.8 percent or 114 patients) were described as "much" and "moderately improved." Further, 138 patients (27.6 percent of the 500) stayed somewhere between 4 to 6 months, and fully 85 percent of these were described as "much" and "moderately

Table 16. Duration of Hospitalization vs. Condition on Discharge

Duration	Much Improved %	Moderately Improved %	Slightly Improved %	Unimproved %	Total %
Less than 1 month	0	5.0	4.0	6.6	15.6
1–3 months	3.6	19.2	4.0	4.0	30.8
4–6 months	5.4	18.0	2.4	1.8	27.6
7–12 months	3.2	9.8	2.6	1.6	17.2
13–24 months	1.4	4.4	0.6	0.2	6.6
Over 24 months	0	1.0	1.0	0.2	2.2
Total	13.6	57.4	14.6	14.4	

improved." Thirty-three patients (6.6 percent of the 500) stayed from 13 to 24 months, and as much as 88 percent of these (29 patients) were described on discharge as "much" and "moderately improved." In other words, the percentage for those patients who stay in hospital treatment 13 to 24 months and who reach the "much" and "moderately improved" level is higher than for those similarly improved patients who stay 1 to 3 months. These statistics are especially significant since they show the decided value of longer-term care. This was shown to be a fact many years ago.[21]

The following facts are notable: (1) a slight majority of the patients (51.2 percent) improve "moderately" and "much" within six months, and more (64.2 percent) do so certainly within one year; (2) however, if patients remain in treatment with us into the second year, the chances percentage-wise (88 percent) for this group to reach the "much" and "moderately improved" level are even better than for the group which stays 1 to 3 months (74 percent). It is apparent that some of these would not have improved sufficiently for discharge with medical consent if they had not stayed more than 12 months; (3) 74 percent of those patients who stay 1 to 3 months are "much" and "moderately improved," 85 percent of those who stay 4 to 6 months reach such levels of improvement, 75 percent of those who stay between 7 to 12 months reach those levels of improvement, and 88 percent of those who stay 13 to 24 months are described in such manner on discharge.

(b) Type of Discharge vs. Condition on Discharge

When one explores the reasons for a patient's discharge at any particular time, he discovers interesting facts to account for the timing. Some of them have been suggested above. Whether

Table 17. Type of Discharge vs. Percentage of Improved and Unimproved

Type of Discharge	Much Improved %	Moderately Improved %	Slightly Improved %	Unimproved %	Total %
With medical approval	9.6	23.2	1.0	0.4	34.2
Against medical approval	4.0	30.0	11.0	10.0	55.0
Other	0	4.6	2.0	4.2	10.8

the patient leaves with or without medical approval seems to be related to his condition upon discharge.

It appears that the condition of patients who are discharged with medical approval is weighted toward much or moderate improvement, while those who leave without such approval are weighted toward moderate to slight improvement or unimprovement. Looking at it another way, approximately the same percentage who are much or moderately improved leave with or without medical approval (32.8 and 34.0 percent). We can only explain this by our apparent conservatism in evaluating patients and our reluctance to see them depart before a really optimal result has been achieved. We stand firm against the removal of patients for "extraneous" reasons.

(c) Diagnosis vs. Type of Discharge

Patients diagnosed Schizophrenia left the hospital without medical approval with the highest incidence (41.6 percent). Psychoneurotic Disorders (9.0 percent) and Personality Disorders (7.8 percent) were next in frequency. Again, this would indicate our cautious approach to the vulnerable schizophrenic and our belief that the hospital should be used to achieve as thorough a result as possible—not a fleeting one.

DISCUSSION

This study was built on a previous one[11] devoted to the various considerations relevant to the evaluation of our clinical work with patients. Contrary to that study, the present article had more in mind the reporting of statistics, which are intended to serve as a basis of comparison with studies already or yet to be done, particularly as these usually emanate from public institutions. Unfortunately, the latter alone act as guides to the profession, which bases its thinking, action, and planning on them. Our additional aim, then, was that this extensive study of 500 cases treated in a proprietary psychiatric hospital, together with other similar ones already or yet to be done, would give the profession a more balanced picture from which to draw its conclusions. It seemed particularly cogent that the demographic and evaluative factors studied might be of use by comparison in community health endeavors, especially those programs which expand the segment of the population treated under them. Beyond this, the study was intended to encourage similar ones. In pursuing such a study one can establish for his own institution valuable procedures for the continuous exploration and standardized assessment of its work with patients. This, of course, was one of our aims for ourselves.

We have attempted to present data about the characteristics of a particular patient population in a particular program with no claim that they should be true for any other group. We have presented the clinical course of our patients and results with them as objectively as possible and irrespective of whether or not the findings reflect favorably on our program. We are aware, too, that the findings hold for a particular period in the lifetime of a hospital and that those for the period 1962–67 might very well be different. As a matter of fact, we are now engaged in another similar study of a recent two-year period with the additional aim of doing a follow-up of the patients so studied. We may be certain that for various reasons the results will differ from those reported here.

The study brought to light factors of which we had been totally unaware. This naturally had a very sobering effect, promoted self-criticism, and led to greater refinement of our clinical work even as we were doing the evaluation. We did not gather statistics, nor do we report them, for their own sake. But the chaff cannot be separated from the wheat until they are known and examined for possible insight into hidden variables that influence our treatment procedures and results. Perhaps, too, they furnish us some better appreciation of factors which play a part in the development and treatment of mental illness generally.

As a result of this study we have become aware that our personal biases and predilections play a part in how we diagnose patients and evaluate their ultimate condition. We found, for instance, that either our hospital attracts a greater percentage of schizophrenics or that we are much freer in diagnosing patients as such than are other hospital psychiatrists. Though we pride ourselves in being "cautiously optimistic" rather than pessimistic about the prognosis for schizophrenics in our care, we did find that we do not think of them as "recovered" as do others and report less of them as "much" improved. Further, we are more reluctant to give them our medical approval for discharge when they themselves or their families think they are well enough to leave our care. Contrary to general belief, however, we did find that long-term care beyond three months, and beyond one year, can lead to good results with schizophrenics who otherwise show no improvement in lesser periods of time. This, too, is significant in view of the current trend to favor and foster short-term hospital or extramural care. However, we do recognize that the durability of remission in patients who received longer-term hospital care has not been adequately compared to that achieved by brief treatment. This is a task yet to be done.

REFERENCES

1. Gralnick, A. "On behavioral determinants in a therapeutic milieu." In *The dynamics of psychiatric drug therapy*. Springfield, Ill.: Thomas, 1959.

2. Gralnick, A., and F. D'Elia. "Role of the patient in the thera-

peutic community: patient participation." *American Journal of Psychotherapy,* 15:63 (1961).

3. Rabiner, E., H. Molinski, and A. Gralnick. "Conjoint family therapy in the inpatient setting." *American Journal of Psychotherapy,* 16:618 (1962).

4. Silverberg, J. W., F. D'Elia, E. Rabiner, and A. Gralnick. "The implementation of psychoanalytic concepts in hospital practice." In *Science and psychoanalysis.* New York: Grune & Stratton, 1964.

5. Rabiner, E., E. Gomez, and A. Gralnick. "The therapeutic community as an insight catalyst." *American Journal of Psychotherapy,* 18:244 (1964).

6. Lind, A., and A. Gralnick. "Integration of the social group worker and psychiatrist in the psychiatric hospital." *International Journal of Social Psychiatry,* 11:53 (1965).

7. Locke, B., M. Kramer, C. Timberlake, B. Pasamanick, and D. Smeltzer. "Problems in interpretation of patterns of first admissions to Ohio state public mental hospitals for patients with schizophrenic reactions." *Psychiatric Research Report 10,* American Psychiatric Association, December 1958, pp. 172–96.

8. Silver, R., and L. Sines. "State hospital and teaching institute treatment results." *Diseases of the Nervous System,* 14:414–19 (1963).

9. Person, P. "Geographic variation in first admission rates to a state mental hospital." *Public Health Reports,* 77:719–31, U.S. Public Health Service, 1962.

10. Pollack, E., R. Redlick, V. Norman, C. Wurster, and K. Gorwitz. "A study of socioeconomic and family characteristics admitted to psychiatric services: background and preliminary analysis." Paper presented at the 90th Annual Meeting of the American Public Health Association, Miami Beach, Fla., October 1962.

11. Greenhill, M., A. Gralnick, R. Duncan, R. Yemez, and F. Turker. "Considerations in evaluating the results of psychotherapy with 500 inpatients." *American Journal of Psychotherapy,* 20:58 (1966).

12. U. S. Department of Health, Education and Welfare. "Patients in mental institutions," part 3, p. 12. Washington, D.C., 1960.

13. *Ibid.,* part 2, p. 39.

14. New York State Department of Mental Hygiene. "Annual report," p. 83. Albany, N.Y., 1960.

15. *Ibid.,* ref. 12, p. 19.

16. *Ibid.,* ref. 14, p. 115.

17. Daniels, R., P. Margolis, and R. Carson. "Hospital discharges

against medical advice." *Archives of General Psychiatry,* 8:120–30 (February 1963).

18. *Ibid.,* pp. 131–38.

19. Greenwald, A., and L. Bartemeier. "Psychiatric discharges against medical advice." *Archives of General Psychiatry,* 8:117–19 (February 1963).

20. New York State, "Annual report," ref. 14, p. 119.

21. Cheney, C., and P. Drewry, Jr. "Results of nonspecific treatment in dementia praecox." *American Journal of Psychiatry,* 95:1 (July 1938).

22. Saarma, J. "Prognosis of insulin therapy in schizophrenia based on higher nervous activity data." *International Journal of Psychiatry,* 2:4 (July 1966).

23. Gralnick, A. "A three-year survey of electroshock therapy." *American Journal of Psychiatry,* 102:5:583–93 (March 1946).

24. Gralnick, A. "A seven-year survey of insulin treatment in schizophrenia." *American Journal of Psychiatry,* 101:4:449–52 (January 1945).

Chapter 15
A Two-year Follow-up of 152
Hospitalized Psychiatric Patients

in collaboration with the senior author, Walmor L. Berger, M.D.

It is natural for psychiatrists, as well as the family, to be concerned with the patient's future. Psychiatrists such as ourselves, who are attached to hospitals, wonder to what extent our particular methods of treatment might be related to the ultimate outcome. Accordingly, we embarked on this follow-up study with such a goal in mind. However, we soon found that as useful a purpose might be served by describing the difficulties we encountered as well as the relatively meager data we could muster.

In searching the literature we were immediately struck with the relatively few comprehensive papers dealing with follow-ups.[1,2,6-12] We found that without an excellent hospital record a good follow-up is relatively useless as a basis of patient comparison. When one makes such a study he really discovers the gross inconsistencies and inadequacies of most records. To guard against this an acceptable and thorough research data form must be attached to each record. Its every item must be understood by the staff and filled in properly.

A major consideration, of course, was what to include in the questionnaire that would give us thoroughness and yet not discourage response nor arouse lingering paranoid reactions which could only distort the data. The initial responses certainly bore out our misgivings. Many patients misinterpreted several of the questions, though these seemed to be so clear and simple to us.

199

Many of the letters, though we ascertained the addresses to be correct, were returned to us or went unanswered. Follow-up letters to these patients did little good. Personal contacts could not be made because of budgetary limitations. Subsequent telephone contacts with these patients disclosed that many had merely consigned the questionnaire to the wastebasket. Some of these patients, however, would respond pleasantly to the questioner. Others, on the other hand, would indicate that they had been "warned" about the matter by other former patients. Their answers, of course, were then quite evasive and paranoid in flavor so that their reliability was questionable. Others indicated a great fear of rehospitalization, and that hospitalization had been a terrible experience which they did not wish to recall. It were as though "The Hospital" actually represented the "bad experience" or frightening psychosis. It was increasingly obvious, too, how really deep-seated was the feeling of stigma about mental illness and that this factor added to our burden in gathering data. Feelings of stigma seemed to be minimized where family therapy had been done or the family seemed to understand and accept the patient. Often the patient's husband would respond quite willingly but indicate that since his wife was doing well he did not want to "remind" her of her illness by showing her the questionnaire.

We received responses to only 26 percent of our letters. However, after numerous telephone calls to the patients, families, friends, and referring psychiatrists, we ended with completed questionnaires on 54 percent of the initial group under study. It is because of the difficulties we encountered that we recommend contact between patient, family, and research team immediately upon hospitalization. Many more responses came from married than from unmarried patients (55 versus 31 percent), though they were rather equally represented in the total group. Otherwise, there seemed to be no essential differences when we matched the various groups which responded.

Setting: High Point Hospital is a proprietary psychiatric hospital which has a bed capacity of 45 and a staff of seven full-time psychiatrists carrying treatment responsibilities. Treatment is based on a dynamic approach, including psychoanalytically oriented psychotherapy for all patients within a therapeutic milieu. Variously included are occupational therapy, activity therapy, family therapy, vocational rehabilitation, and drugs and electroconvulsive therapy whenever indicated. Each patient receives three full sessions of psychotherapy per week. In our treatment program the patient is placed in a group system in which he is moved according to his capacity to tolerate greater contact with other patients and also to assume greater responsibility within the hospital community. The groups are numbered from I to IV, the latter being that group in which the patient has the most "freedom" but also the most responsibility within the hospital community. The program has been described in greater detail in other publications.[3-5]

CHARACTERISTICS AT DISCHARGE OF THE STUDY POPULATION

This study includes all patients admitted to High Point Hospital during the years of 1964–65, making a total of 166. The main characteristic of this study group can be seen in the data that follows:

The average age of our patients was 32.3 years; for the females it was 35.2 and for the males, 29.3 years. The average for patients under 21 was 17.3 years. The average length of stay was 152 days.

Previous Hospitalization

Fifty-nine percent of our patients had been hospitalized before; 31 percent of them had more than one hospitalization. Of the patients ill more than 11 years, only 15 percent had not been in a psychiatric hospital before.

Length of Hospitalization

In our group system, patients of a higher group generally have been in the hospital for a longer period of time. The average length of stay for the Group IV patients was 210 days and for the other groups, 188, 94, and 172 days, respectively for Groups III,

II, and I. Patients who had had no previous psychiatric treatment had a shorter (112 days) stay in the hospital than those who had had ambulatory treatment (123 days) or previous hospitalization (156 days). Diagnostically, nonschizophrenic patients had a much shorter (98 days) stay than those diagnosed "schizophrenic reaction" (152 days). Within this last group, length of stay varied from 45 to 442 days in the following order: acute undifferentiated (45 days), catatonic (109 days), simple (120 days), paranoid (146 days), chronic undifferentiated (151 days), schizo-affective (168 days), mixed (304 days), and hebephrenic (442 days).

Procedure

The medical records of 166 patients were carefully reviewed and evaluated. Identifying data and information about the patient's past history were given in detail on our research data forms. Special attention was given to the level of functioning that the patient had reached in the hospital, as well as to his condition on discharge and the different factors which could have resulted in any patient's premature discharge.

The follow-up was done with the help of a questionnaire that was sent to all the patients. Each form took the patient's admission number and gave each patient the chance to sign it only if he wished. The questionnaire contained 21 items, including inquiries into the following: Current psychiatric treatment, type of treatment (psychotherapy or medication), how he spent most of his time (at home, job, or school), his employment history, his adjustment at school, how he used his spare time, social activities, organizational memberships, recurrence of symptoms, all subsequent hospitalizations (reasons for readmissions and treatment), his physical health, and how the hospitalization had affected his life. Whenever necessary we contacted the referring physician to learn more about the patient's adjustment in the community.

One of our most difficult problems was establishing standards by which to evaluate the adjustment of the patient on the basis of the data obtained from him and others. Getting information was always an easier task when the interviewer knew the person he was contacting. In several situations even the refer-ring physician seemed cautious in revealing data about his patient, but generally we were able to get data that seemed sufficient to confirm or deny what the patient had revealed.

We considered a patient as functioning well or making a good adjustment if he had a steady occupation (job, study, house-work) and otherwise engaged in normal family life. We inquired into what he did with his spare time. Did he engage in and enjoy reading, listening to music, playing the piano, gardening, camp-ing, etc. We also expected such patients to have some social life and activities away from home. We found that many patients acquired hobbies while in the hospital that they kept enjoying after discharge. We considered a patient as making a "fair adjustment" if he worked and said he passed his spare time in reading and watching TV but had "no social life." One house-wife said that her weekend was a "housewife's weekend" and that in her spare time she read her Bible. We classified her as making a "fair adjustment." We classified as "marginal" all patients reporting abundant symptomatology. We realize that these criteria for judgment are very loose and that some patients classified as having made a fair adjustment within their family context or way of life might have been doing well, or by the same token, very poorly.

Posthospital Adaptation

Of the original 166 patients admitted in 1964 and 1965, three yet remained hospitalized with us, and 11 had been transferred to other institutions, and, therefore, not followed: Essentially, then, we followed 152 patients who had been discharged from our care and obtained information on 75 of these sufficient to make some judgment about their adjustment. Three patients committed suicide after an average of four months. Another was killed while driving an automobile, which we tended to accept as a suicide because he had made two serious attempts on his life prior to hospitalization. These four deaths by suicide would make 2.6 percent of the 152 followed.

Of the 75 responding patients, 43 were in treatment at the time of the survey (1966–67). The majority (27) were in psy-

chotherapy and on some medication, while 10 were in psychotherapy alone. Fifty-eight of the 75 were involved in productive
activity that may be described as follows: adequate functioning
as housewives supplemented by part-time work or study; full-
time work or full-time study; or part-time work supplemented by
part-time study. Patients who went from job to job generally
ended up rehospitalized.

Forty-one of the patients reporting experienced some recurrence of symptoms, and 20 percent were rehospitalized within the
period of the study. Single patients were rehospitalized three
times more frequently than married ones. In most instances
patients who were rehospitalized had been discharged against
medical advice. Although patients in their twenties composed
about 20 percent of the group studied, they composed about 50
percent of those who were rehospitalized. Forty-three of the 75
patients made what appeared to be a good to very good adjustment, and 11 a fair adaptation. The remainder were "marginal."
The average follow-up time was 18 months.

Apparently "higher education" plays a role in the nature of
the patient's posthospital adjustment. College students and graduates made up 90 percent of those who made a "very good"
adjustment in the community, and a major percentage of those
who made a "good" adjustment. Patients who had not completed high school were a major percentage of those who made a
"marginal" adjustment.

The religion of the patients seemed to bear no relationship to
the type of adjustment made after hospitalization. However, the
duration of illness before hospitalization did seem to be related
to the quality of the later adjustment. Only 25 percent of the
patients who had been ill for several years or more made a good
adjustment. The greatest majority of these had left the hospital
against medical advice. On the other hand, an average of 70
percent of those ill for shorter periods of time made a good
adjustment after discharge. Of the 11 patients judged to have
made a "very good" adjustment, 10 had reached the Group IV
level in the hospital and had been discharged as "improved" and
"very much improved." In this group they had the longest
average period of hospitalization

SUMMARY AND CONCLUSIONS

The patients had been admitted in 1964 and 1965, and the average follow-up time was one and one-half years. The questionnaire covered some 21 items meant to elicit information on which a fairly accurate judgment could be made of the patient's posthospital adjustment. From the information obtained, patients' adjustment was judged as "marginal" to "fair to good" and finally "very good." Some relatively elastic standards were established upon which to base these judgments.

Information was obtained from about 50 percent of those we had sought to contact. This is not a very good percentage. Short of following the very expensive procedure of sending personal envoys to see patients and relatives, we suggest that the percentage of returns could be raised. This might be achieved by having the research team become acquainted with the patient and family immediately upon hospitalization and remain so throughout the patient's stay. In this manner the study and follow-up could be seen as part and parcel of the entire treatment process intended for the patient's welfare.

BIBLIOGRAPHY

1. Bucove, A. D., and L. I. Levitt. "A seven-year follow-up study of patients in a general hospital psychiatric service." *American Journal of Psychiatry,* 122:1088–95, 1096.

2. Cole, N. J., B. W. McDonald, and C. H. H. Branch. "A two-year follow-up study of the work performance of former psychiatric patients." *American Journal of Psychiatry,* 124:8 (February 1968).

3. Greenhill, M. H., A. Gralnick, R. H. Duncan, R. Yemez, and F. Turker. "Considerations in evaluating the results of psychotherapy with 500 inpatients." *American Journal of Psychotherapy,* 20:1:58–68 (January 1966).

4. Gralnick, A., R. Yemez, F. Turker, P. Schween, and M. H. Greenhill. "Five hundred case study in a private psychiatric hospital: further considerations in evaluation." *New York State Psychiatric Quarterly,* forthcoming.

5. Gralnick, A., E. L. Rabiner, G. Del Castillo, and D. Zawel. "The

adolescent inpatient: treatment considerations and report on ninety-two cases.'' Manuscript.

6. Levenstein, S., D. F. Klein, and M. Pollack. "Follow-up study of formerly hospitalized psychiatric patients: the first two years.'' *American Journal of Psychiatry,* 122:10 (April 1966).

7. May, P. R. A., A. H. Tuma, and W. Kraude. "Community follow-up of treatment of schizophrenia—issues and problems.'' *American Journal of Orthopsychiatry,* 35:4 (July 1965).

8. Rassidakis, N. C., C. Lykas, E. Papadakis, and A. Kafatou. "A follow-up study of schizophrenic patients: relapse and readmission.'' *B. Menninger Clinic,* 27:1 (January 1963).

9. Schooler, N. R., S. C. Goldberg, H. Boother, and J. O. Colr. "One year after discharge: community adjustment of schizophrenic patients.'' *American Journal of Psychiatry,* 123:8 (February 1967).

10. Sinnett, E. R., W. E. Stimpert, and E. Straight. "A five-year follow-up study of psychiatric patients.'' *American Journal of Orthopsychiatry,* 35:3 (April 1965).

11. Smith, C. M., and A. B. Levey. "The follow-up study in psychiatry.'' *Diseases of the Nervous System,* 27:595–99 (September 1966).

12. Wilder, J. F., G. Levin, and I. Azerling. "A two-year follow-up evaluation of acute psychotic patients treated in a day hospital.'' *American Journal of Psychiatry,* 122:10 (April 1966).

Chapter 16
Leadership Effect on the Staff Conference Process

Leatrice Styrt Schacht, M.A., and Murray Blacker, Ph.D.

In recent years increasing attention has been given to the total context in which hospital treatment is applied. Social scientists have been brought into hospital settings to help study and define the forces operating within the psychotherapeutic field which influence staff attitudes and decision-making in regard to patients. Concurrent with this has been the advent of the concept of the therapeutic community which has been received and applied with considerable enthusiasm. In such a community the course of treatment is particularly influenced by a complex network of interrelationships. The studies of Stanton and Schwartz,[1] Caudill,[2] and others have served to emphasize the importance and broaden the understanding of how the structure and communication system among the personnel in the hospital affects the therapeutic process. These researchers emphasize the need to direct attention to the specific identification of special patterns of interaction among the personnel because so much remains that is far from explicit as to how therapeutic community concepts and procedures ameliorate psychopathology.

This study may help in the understanding of how certain senior authorities of a hospital affect the forces operating within the therapeutic field. Some research reports have attended to the role of the higher administrative authorities in such settings[3]; but relatively less attention has been paid to the specifics of how

207

decision-making and staff attitudes are affected by the interaction between such authorities and the doctor responsible for the care of the individual patient. Our study deals, in particular, with the staff clinical-administrative conference and is the outgrowth of the observations by two independent psychologists of 61 weekly meetings of the psychiatric staff of a 45-bed treatment hospital devoted to intensive psychotherapy within a well-established therapeutic community organization. The operational organization of High Point Hospital has been described elsewhere.[4,5]

It is pertinent to point out that the general atmosphere is that of a highly integrated therapeutic community with patient participation in group meetings and hospital activities, in addition to three individual hours of psychotherapy weekly. Most patients carry the diagnosis of schizophrenia and are hospitalized for many months, so that a sense of continuity is maintained.

The staff conferences were held weekly. Each lasted over three hours and centered on major reviews and changes in patient status. The therapists were expected to discuss in brief the ongoing situation of each patient and to vote on all administrative-treatment decisions, including hospital privileges, home visits, program changes, and medication at this meeting. It assumed, therefore, a central and crucial role in the social and treatment process of the hospital.

The two independent observers attended these conferences as part of a larger research study on doctor-patient tensions.* This was, in essence, a multiobservational approach to the study of doctor-patient relationships within a hospital setting. The weekly staff meeting was one of the observation points. The observers' job was to judge and rate the tensions generated by the staff interaction which might then be carried back into the individual therapy sessions. The data sheet (Staff Meeting Rating Form), which follows the regular form the staff discussions took, was used to record the ratings. Adequate inter-rater relia-

*Doctor-Patient Tensions: Their Measurement and Relationship to Outcome. This five-year research project was jointly supported by the USPHS (grants No. MO-05392 and MH-08018) and The Gralnick Foundation.

Staff Meeting Rating Form   High Point Hospital

Patient _____Therapist _____Rater _____

I Therapist Report   Dates
  A. Clinical Course
    1 Marked improvement   ☐☐☐☐☐☐
    2 Slight improvement   ☐☐☐☐☐☐
    3 No change   ☐☐☐☐☐☐
    4 Slightly worse   ☐☐☐☐☐☐
    5 Markedly worse   ☐☐☐☐☐☐
  B. Progress of Psychotherapy
    1 Patient producing
      meaningful material   ☐☐☐☐☐☐
    2 No meaningful material   ☐☐☐☐☐☐
    3 Direction of therapeutic
      movement (+ or −)   ☐☐☐☐☐☐
    4 Rapport with doctor
      (+ or −)   ☐☐☐☐☐☐
  C. Tension Indicators
      (rated on a scale 0-2)
    1 Patient complaining   ☐☐☐☐☐☐
    2 Patient dissatisfied
      with privileges   ☐☐☐☐☐☐
    3 Patient distrusts therapist   ☐☐☐☐☐☐

    4 Patient angry at therapist   ☐☐☐☐☐☐
    5 Patient requests change
      of therapist   ☐☐☐☐☐☐
    6 Patient wants to leave
      hospital   ☐☐☐☐☐☐
    7 Family pressuring therapist   ☐☐☐☐☐☐
    8 Referring doctor pressuring
      therapist   ☐☐☐☐☐☐

  D. Therapist's Attitude
    1 Openly enthusiastic   ☐☐☐☐☐☐
    2 Interested   ☐☐☐☐☐☐
    3 Neutral   ☐☐☐☐☐☐
    4 Discouraged   ☐☐☐☐☐☐
    5 Feels bored or burdened   ☐☐☐☐☐☐

II Staff Reaction
    1 Minimum interaction   ☐☐☐☐☐☐
    2 Therapist asked to clarify
      or enlarge report   ☐☐☐☐☐☐
    3 Reassuring comments
      from staff   ☐☐☐☐☐☐

Staff Meeting Rating Form—High Point Hospital

Patient _____Therapist _____Rater _____

III Changes in Patient's Program   Dates
  A. Direction of Initiative
    for Change
    1 Number of therapist's
      request   ☐☐☐☐☐☐
    2 Number of therapist's requests
      rejected   ☐☐☐☐☐☐
    3 Number of requests initiated
      by staff   ☐☐☐☐☐☐
    4 Number of therapist's requests
      carried over therapist's
      Objections   ☐☐☐☐☐☐
  B. Timing
    1 Staff more cautious than
      therapist   ☐☐☐☐☐☐
    2 Staff less cautious than
      therapist   ☐☐☐☐☐☐
  C. Impact of Interaction Between
    Staff & Therapist
    1 Therapist's concern re: patient
      greater (+) less (−)   ☐☐☐☐☐☐
    2 Therapist's concern re: himself
      greater (+) less (−)   ☐☐☐☐☐☐

    3 Staff critical of management
      of patient (rated on
      a scale 1-3)   ☐☐☐☐☐☐
    4 Open clash
      (specify with whom)   ☐☐☐☐☐☐
      (a.) Rate on a scale 1-3   ☐☐☐☐☐☐
IV Therapist's Behavior
    1 Takes no stand   ☐☐☐☐☐☐
    2 Assertive (rate on scale
      1 to 3+)   ☐☐☐☐☐☐
    3 Accepts   ☐☐☐☐☐☐
    4 Submits   ☐☐☐☐☐☐
    5 Tension level (TL)
      (rate on scale 0-2)   ☐☐☐☐☐☐
      (a.) TL greater than   ☐☐☐☐☐☐
      warranted by interaction   ☐☐☐☐☐☐
      (b.) TL appropriate to
      interaction   ☐☐☐☐☐☐
      (c.) TL less than warranted
      by interaction   ☐☐☐☐☐☐
V Unusual Responses
    (check and describe
    reverse side)   ☐☐☐☐☐☐

bility was obtained and refinement of the instrument was established through a series of trial forms and runs.

The meetings were most often headed by the clinical director (Dr. B) with the staff of six psychiatric residents and the chief nurse in regular attendance. The head of the hospital (Dr. A) also attended, but he was sometimes absent for protracted periods. When the clinical director was not present, Dr. A took over the running of the meetings.

The observers had noted early in their attendance at these staff conferences that there was a marked difference in interaction between staff and leader depending on who was leader. This had been emphasized in the summary notes customarily made after each conference.

SAMPLE

Sample comments in summary notes—Dr. B leading conferences.

(1) "Meeting really a discussion of management details rather than patients."

(2) "Obsession with irrelevant details pervades meeting."

(3) "Feeling of boredom, stress appears to be on control of patients."

Dr. A leading conference.

(1) "Conference somewhat more alive, more pointed, more goal-directed."

(2) "Problems of communication among medical staff discussed."

(3) "Impression is that Dr. A is more clearly involved with resident's case loads with resulting sense of support and cooperation."

It was hypothesized that the data of the staff meetings would evidence significant differences related to which leader was conducting the conference. It was expected that the differences would be in the direction of showing greater and more positive interaction with Dr. A conducting the conferences.

An opportunity to test this out was provided by the fact that there was one consecutive block of time when Dr. B was leading the conferences (toward the beginning of the time period of research observation), and another consecutive block of time when Dr. A was leading the conferences (toward the end of the period of observation). Thus it was hoped that a difference seen throughout the observation period could be brought into sharp

Table 1. Description of Patient Discussions During Two Periods of Different Staff Conference Leaders

Doctor	No. Conferences Led	No. Patients Discussed	Total Patient Discussions	Mean No. Patient Discussions
B	18	75	685	9.49
A	12	41	389	9.13
Total	30	116	1,074	

focus by comparing data sheet material for these two demarcated time periods.

Although the period of Dr. B's separate leadership was longer than the period for Dr. A, there was no difference between the mean number of patients discussed during each time period. Table 1 describes the number of conferences, number of patients discussed, total number of patient discussions, and the mean number of patients discussed during the two time periods.

RESULTS

The summary of the findings is described in Table 2. Many items on the data sheet were only infrequently checked, making them not useful for statistical study, and they were thus eliminated. Other items that occurred on a continuum (clinical course, therapist's attitude) were infrequently checked at the extremes and for statistical purposes were condensed into a smaller group. Statistical procedures were applied as appropriate, using χ^2 and the t-test.

An examination of Table 2 indicates that three aspects of the therapist's report (category I-A, B, D)* were significantly differ-

Table 2. Summary of Findings

Rating Form Items Studied	Statistical Result	Probability (Significance)
I Therapist Report		
A. *Clinical Course*		
1 & 2 Markedly and slightly improved		
3 No change	$\chi^2 = 16.71$	<0.001
4 & 5 Slightly and markedly worse		
B. *Progress of Psychotherapy*		
1 Patient producing meaningful material	$t = 2.59$	<0.05
C. *Tension Indicators** (all categories 1–8)	$t = 1.40$	ns
D. *Therapist's Attitude*		
1 & 2 Openly enthusiastic and interested		
3 Neutral	$\chi^2 = 38.34$	<0.001
4 & 5 Discouraged and feels bored or burdened		
II Staff Reaction†		
1 Minimum interaction	$t = 4.48$	<0.01
2 Staff asks therapist to clarify or enlarge report	$t = 1.45$	ns
3 Reassuring comments from staff	$t = 2.69$	<0.01
III Changes in Patient's Program		
A. *Direction of Initiative for Change*		
1 No. of therapist's requests	$t = 2.30$	<0.05
1 & 2 No. of therapist's requests minus those rejected	$\chi^2 = 209$	ns
3 No. of requests initiated by staff	$t = 4.70$	<0.01
B. *Timing‡*		
1 Staff more cautious than therapist	$t = 2.03$	0.05
C. *Impact of Interaction Between Staff and Therapist*		
1 Therapist's concern regarding patient increased (+)	$t = 0.09$	ns
2 Therapist's concern regarding himself increased (+)	$t = 0.81$	ns
IV Therapist's Behavior		
2 Assertive	$t = 1.41$	ns
1, 3 & 4 Takes no stand, accepts and/or submits	$t = 0.38$	ns
5 Tension level	$t = 0.70$	ns

*Category C showed significant difference when an F-test was used indicating that the range of tension indicators checked was greater with Dr. B. in charge. An analysis of the breakdown of the various Tension Indicators, which for the purposes of this study were all lumped together, might have yielded more specific differences (but was not feasible owing to the limited number of entries).

†Staff refers to any member of the conference other than the presenting resident. Unfortunately no provision on the data sheet was made to differentiate between the leader and other staff members. However, it was clinically observed that staff reaction more often came from the leader.

‡Cautioning statements are illustrated by such remarks as "Let's wait and see if he really settles down"; "Perhaps he's trying to manipulate you"; "In my experience you can't count on—————."

ent when Dr. A was in charge. With Dr. A the resident more frequently reported his patient as being improved (I-A), as producing meaningful material in psychotherapy (I-B), and as eliciting a more positive attitude from his therapist (I-D). With Dr. B, the therapist's report was significantly more negative in relation to all these variables.

In Category II (Staff Reaction)† Minimum Interaction (II-1) was significantly higher with Dr. B in charge. Minimum Interaction refers either to a neutral "no change" for the residents' report without any requests or questions being asked, or a general lack of reaction to the residents' report. No significant difference between the two leaders was found in requests by the staff that the residents' report be clarified or enlarged (II-2), whereas there was significantly more reassuring comments from the staff (II-3) with Dr. A in charge.

In Category III (Changes in Patient's Program) no significant difference occurred as to the number of therapist requests accepted or rejected (III-A2), but requests made by the staff (III-A3) and requests made by the therapist (III-A1) were significantly higher when Dr. A was leading.

In the items under Timing (III-B) the degree to which the staff cautioned‡ the therapist (III-B1) was significantly higher with Dr. A in charge. In the remaining items in Category III (III-B2, III-C1 and 2) no significant differences appeared, nor were there any significant differences in any of the measures of Category IV (Therapists' Behavior).

COMMENT

The most significant finding of this study was that the differences in the quality of the staff interaction under the leadership of the two different heads could be measured objectively. The hypothesis to be tested was arrived at only after a long period of observation. It was only at this point that a careful perusal of the summary notes to substantiate clinical impression crystallized the notion that these measures might be forthcoming even though the instrument itself was not intended or designed as such a predictive device.

The next important findings were in the specific areas in which the different leaders affected the course of the conferences. The initial spontaneous residents' report was markedly influenced by the presence of a particular leader. One could only assume that there was an expectation of a certain reaction from the two leaders. For example, it could be hypothesized that if the therapist painted a positive picture of his patient, he could get more privileges for him. However, an examination of the number of requests granted (III-A1) shows that there is no significant difference in the number of requests accepted when Dr. A is leading or when Dr. B is leading, this despite the fact that Dr. A had greater final authority as head of the hospital to grant or reject requests.

An examination of findings for Category II (Staff Reaction) gives a clue to one of the major differences between the leaders and their reaction to the therapist's report. With Dr. A leading, there were significantly fewer times when the discussion of the patient ended because there was "a minimum of interaction." When minimum interaction was checked, the most likely therapist's report had been a bland, neutral "no change." No request would be made or response expected. There was no significant difference between the two leaders in asking the therapist to clarify or enlarge his report. Thus the therapist's report was apparently taken at face value. Actually, this also might indicate a considerable autonomy on the part of the therapist. (This is borne out by the researchers' observation that in this hospital about 80 percent of the therapists' requests are granted.) It is then even more interesting that with that amount of autonomy the residents reported so differently when the different leaders presided. That there were significantly more reassuring comments from the staff when Dr. A led is consonant with the more positive atmosphere of the therapists' report under his leadership.

The results of studying Category III (Changes in the Patient's Program) again direct attention to the interaction between leader and therapist. Although there was no significant difference between the two leaders when considering the number of therapist's requests accepted, there were significantly more requests made by the therapist and significantly more requests made by the staff when Dr. A was leading. It is interesting that with Dr. A leading there is significantly more caution on the part of the staff. Probably this parallels the fact that more reassuring comments were made when he was leading. In other words, the interaction was less cut and dried—more activity was seen, whether in the form of therapist's request, staff request, reassuring comments, or expression of caution.

One then comes to a crucial question—does more active leadership relate to a more positive therapist-patient approach? From this study that would seem to be true. An interesting parallel question arises. We know here that under active leadership, the therapist more often perceives his patient as getting better. A study to answer whether there is an actual difference in improvement rates under such conditions would be indicated.

The original study on Doctor-Patient Tensions was spurred by a hypothesis that the staff conference might leave a residue of tension that would result in hampering the doctor-patient relationship. Direct results of our study do not indicate significant differences in Therapists' Reactions and Behavior (Category IV) when one or the other leader is present. (The direction, however, is for more residual tension when Dr. B leads conference.) Thus our findings appear to be that it is in the area of the therapist's perception of his patient and in the interaction between therapist and leader that there are the greatest differences. Work in process, evaluating the behavior of the residents as a group over the entire time period regardless of leadership factors, indicates a clustering of factors in the behavior of the therapists that is undoubtedly related to our findings here. For example, there is a very high correlation between the therapist seeing his patient improved, making more requests, being more assertive, and being more positive in his attitude toward the patient. Thus, perhaps a leader who elicits a more positive response from his residents may set off a whole chain of responses related to the patient's course of treatment.

With Dr. A in charge, the staff made statistically significant moves toward more openness and more involvement with what was being discussed. The difference with the clinical director in charge appeared to be that the meetings were more managerial, with an emphasis on control and domination, whereas with the head of the hospital there was more willingness to interchange ideas and feelings. Gibb [6(p94)] states that the "concept of domination and headship is important because it is so different from that of leadership, and because so much so-called leadership in industry, education, and in other social spheres is not leadership at all, but is simply domination. It is not, however, necessary that domination should preclude leadership.''

The ideal mode of relatedness at the conferences could be said to be an emphasis on consciousness of communication which would take into account the inner, subjective meanings and would avoid dogmatic objectivity. The problems discussed were expected to be settled by staff consensus. Any resolution had to be consistent with the many written regulations and rules provided for the highly organized therapeutic community structure. There was a stress on social interaction for both patients and staff within firm but flexible limits, and with clear lines of authority and responsibility.

The impression from the statistics and observations is that the conferences functioned more in line with the hospital's ideology when the head of the hospital was the leader. He was the final arbiter and implementor of the principles on which the hospital operated, and he was clearly the dominant figure at the conferences. The trend of the conferences was toward covertness, rigidity, and authoritarianism when the clinical director (Dr. B) was in charge. An important reason for this may have been that the head of the hospital (Dr. A) had more of the genuine power. The clinical director also had power which was delegated to him—but may not have functioned so closely in line with the hospital ideology. This could be readily sensed at the meetings. When the head of the hospital was leading, the atmosphere was one of alertness and anticipation that significant issues would be dealt with and resolved. With the clinical director, an obsessive attention to irrelevant details and a sense of boredom were more often noted. The result was a muddling of communication which depressed the possibility of openness of interchange at the meetings.

Another aspect of power has to do with the residents' willingness to abrogate their power at these meetings. This seemed more prevalent with the clinical director in charge. In a conference with the head of the hospital after the period of observations had ended, he pointed out that he had to actively encourage the residents toward more participation. Rubenstein and

Lasswell[3] tend to confirm this. In their study they had the residents complete questionnaires in which they indicated that they were only too willing to accept the superior power of their seniors "asking only that they be cared for and respected."

This staff clinical-administrative conference was formed for the purpose of disseminating information and for decision-making. Whoever was in charge had to direct the meeting toward settling immediate and often urgent problems. The fact that about 80 percent of the therapists' requests were granted indicates that this was generally accomplished. In a related study Caudill[2(p297)] reports that the residents had slightly less than a 50 percent chance for gaining what they had requested. Perhaps one of the reasons for the higher percentage of requests granted at High Point Hospital was that the classical therapist-administrator split described elsewhere[1,2] did not hold. Studies of small groups[7] seem to indicate that these two functions in the hands of a single individual are very difficult to carry out. Yet Stanton and Schwartz and Caudill report dramatic incidents where this split in function engendered its own problem and seriously interfered with the decision-making process.

Another possible reason why decision-making at this conference was relatively enhanced could be that only two levels of authority were involved—the head of the meeting and the residents. This is more in line with efficient industrial conferences rather than those described in the various studies of mental hospitals. Etzione[8(p21)] points out the confusions resulting from therapeutic community administrative conferences where many levels of authority participate. Such conferences are reported to serve more as a source of anxiety than as a positive influence.

SUMMARY

A study by two observers describes the influence of two different leaders of staff conferences on the resident's perception of and report on his patients' progress. Thus the significant role senior staff leadership may have in the doctor's perception of his patients is delineated. It seemed to the observers that the leader who clearly engaged in a more active expression of the hospital philosophy facilitated more positive interaction and openness with the group. This was demonstrated by a statistical study of staff conference data. Thus the more effective leader may have furthered the possibility of bringing this positive attitude into the individual doctor-patient treatment setting.

The implications of these findings for further research lie in two major areas:

1. Exploration of how active leadership relates to a more positive therapist-patient approach and study of whether there are actual differences in patient improvement rates under positive leadership conditions.

2. In residency training programs the main area explored is often the relationship between the doctor (and other health personnel) and the patient. Clinical conferences generally rely heavily on such data for educational purposes. However, the staff relationship, particularly that of conference leader and residents, may play a much more critical role than previously realized and deserve much more detailed examination.

The statistical consultation and subsequent analyses were performed by Daniel Zawel.

REFERENCES

1. Stanton, A. H., and M. S. Schwartz. *The mental hospital.* New York: Basic Books, 1954.

2. Caudill, W. *The psychiatric hospital as a small society.* Cambridge, Mass.: Harvard Univ. Press, 1958.

3. Rubenstein, R., and H. Lasswell. *The sharing of power in a psychiatric hospital.* New Haven: Yale Univ. Press, 1966.

4. Gralnick, A., and F. D'Elia. "Role of the patient in the therapeutic community." *American Journal of Psychotherapy,* 15:63–72 (January 1961).

5. Rabiner, E., E. Gomez, and A. Gralnick. "The therapeutic community as an insight catalyst." *American Journal of Psychotherapy,* 18:244–58 (April 1964).

6. Gibb, C. A. "The principles and traits of leadership." *Abnormal Social Psychology,* 42:267–84 (April 1947).

7. Bales, R. F. *Interaction process analysis.* Cambridge, Mass.: Addison-Wesley, 1950.

8. Etzione, A. "Impersonal and structural factors in the study of mental hospitals." *Psychiatry,* 23:13–22 (February 1960).

Chapter 17
Activity Patterns of Psychiatric
Residents at a Staff Conference

Murray Blacker, Ph.D., and Leatrice Styrt Schacht,
M.A.

The staff conference in a psychiatric hospital with a therapeutic
community organization can and should be a key point in the
hospital's decision-making and communications system. It is
expected to be modeled in a relatively open and democratic form
in which decisions can be made by the group and in which
information can be shared in a way which helps eliminate unnecessary anxiety. However, social scientists such as Stanton and
Schwartz[1] and Caudill,[2] who have reported extensively on the
functioning of staff conferences, indicated that these meetings
were too often negative in their effect. Etzione,[3] in his percep-
tive critical discussion of mental hospital researches, came to
the conclusion that the conferences were too often manipulative
and unnecessarily anxiety-arousing. He questioned whether the
staff really participated in the decision-making process. Evi-
dently much has to be clarified about the functioning of such
meetings in order to help make them more effective instruments
in carrying out the treatment philosophy inherent in the concept
of a therapeutic community.

As members of a research team involved in a multiobservational approach to the study of doctor-patient* relationships, we

*Doctor-Patient Tensions: Their Measurement and Relationship to Out-
come. This five-year research project was jointly supported by the Public
Health Service (grants MO-05392 and MH-08018) and The Gralnick Foundation.

had an opportunity to observe staff activity at conferences over an extended period. We attended 61 consecutive, weekly clinical-administrative conferences at a 45-bed psychiatric hospital with a well-established structured therapeutic community organization. The operational organization of High Point Hospital has been described elsewhere.[4] Our job was to rate tensions generated in individual psychiatric residents by staff interaction which might be carried back into individual therapy sessions with patients. In the course of their experience at the conferences, the observers became interested in more than final tension scores. They noted a relationship between a resident's behavior, perception of his patients, and conference leadership. A study of the influence of two different leaders was reported on in a separate paper.[5] We also observed a patterning of the residents' activity which seemed to have a consistency of its own regardless of the conference leaders. This communication deals with a statistical study of, as well as clinical implications of, this type of patterning. Because of the small sample, it is, in effect, a pilot study of the details of the residents' activity at the meeting. The purpose is to work toward understanding more about the behavior elicited by a conference of this type, how patterns emerge, and what meaning they might have in terms of the efficacy of the conference.

These staff conferences were scheduled for a three-hour period weekly and were reserved for major reviews and negotiations for changes of patients' status. In regular attendance were six psychiatric residents, the chief nurse, and the clinical director and/or the medical director. The meetings generally opened with a brief discussion of the emotional tone of the hospital. Then each patient was discussed in turn, beginning with a statement by the therapist as to the patient's progress over the week in the hospital milieu and in psychotherapy. Other staff members contributed relevant observations. Nursing notes were funneled through the head nurse to the staff at this point. The therapist might then request privileges and program changes which he felt were appropriate to the ongoing therapeutic goals for his patient. It was expected and often asked of the therapist that he be quite explicit about the combined therapeutic and administrative rea-

Staff Meeting Rating Form—High Point Hospital

Patient _____Therapist _____Rater _____

I Therapist Report   Dates
  A. *Clinical Course*
    1 Marked improvement   ☐☐☐☐☐☐
    2 Slight improvement   ☐☐☐☐☐☐
    3 No change   ☐☐☐☐☐☐
    4 Slightly worse   ☐☐☐☐☐☐
    5 Markedly worse   ☐☐☐☐☐☐
  B. *Progress of Psychotherapy*
    1 Patient producing
      meaningful material   ☐☐☐☐☐☐
    2 No meaningful material   ☐☐☐☐☐☐
    3 Direction of therapeutic
      movement (+ or −)   ☐☐☐☐☐☐
    4 Rapport with doctor
      (+ or −)   ☐☐☐☐☐☐
  C. *Tension Indicators*
    (rated on a scale 0-2)
    1 Patient complaining   ☐☐☐☐☐☐
    2 Patient dissatisfied
      with privileges   ☐☐☐☐☐☐
    3 Patient distrusts therapist   ☐☐☐☐☐☐
    4 Patient angry at therapist   ☐☐☐☐☐☐
    5 Patient requests change
      of therapist   ☐☐☐☐☐☐
    6 Patient wants to leave
      hospital   ☐☐☐☐☐☐
    7 Family pressuring therapist   ☐☐☐☐☐☐
    8 Referring doctor pressuring
      therapist   ☐☐☐☐☐☐
  D. *Therapist's Attitude*
    1 Openly enthusiastic   ☐☐☐☐☐☐
    2 Interested   ☐☐☐☐☐☐
    3 Neutral   ☐☐☐☐☐☐
    4 Discouraged   ☐☐☐☐☐☐
    5 Feels bored or burdened   ☐☐☐☐☐☐

II Staff Reaction
    1 Minimum interaction   ☐☐☐☐☐☐
    2 Therapist asked to clarify
      or enlarge report   ☐☐☐☐☐☐
    3 Reassuring comments
      from staff   ☐☐☐☐☐☐

III Changes in Patient's Program   Dates
  A. *Direction of Initiative*
    for Change
    1 Number of therapist's
      request   ☐☐☐☐☐☐
    2 Number of therapist's requests
      rejected   ☐☐☐☐☐☐
    3 Number of requests initiated
      by staff   ☐☐☐☐☐☐
    4 Number of therapist's requests
      carried over therapist's
      Objections   ☐☐☐☐☐☐
  B. *Timing*
    1 Staff more cautious than
      therapist   ☐☐☐☐☐☐
    2 Staff less cautious than
      therapist   ☐☐☐☐☐☐
  C. *Impact of Interaction Between*
    Staff & Therapist
    1 Therapist's concern re: patient
      greater (+) less (−)   ☐☐☐☐☐☐
    2 Therapist's concern re: himself
      greater (+) less (−)   ☐☐☐☐☐☐
    3 Staff critical of management
      of patient (rated on
      a scale 1-3)   ☐☐☐☐☐☐
    4 Open clash
      (specify with whom)   ☐☐☐☐☐☐
      (a.) Rate on a scale 1-3   ☐☐☐☐☐☐

IV Therapist's Behavior
    1 Takes no stand   ☐☐☐☐☐☐
    2 Assertive (rate on scale
      1 to 3+)   ☐☐☐☐☐☐
    3 Accepts   ☐☐☐☐☐☐
    4 Submits   ☐☐☐☐☐☐
    5 Tension level (TL)
      (rate on scale 0-2)   ☐☐☐☐☐☐
      (a.) TL greater than
      warranted by interaction   ☐☐☐☐☐☐
      (b.) TL appropriate to
      interaction   ☐☐☐☐☐☐
      (c.) TL less than warranted
      by interaction   ☐☐☐☐☐☐

V Unusual Responses
  (check and describe
  reverse side)   ☐☐☐☐☐☐

sons for any proposed change. Therefore much of what he said was colored by his concern about his request being granted (and it was thought that much of the tension he might carry out of the staff meeting could be based on his lack of success in justifying what he wanted for his patient). Staff discussion of these requests—sometimes vigorous and heated—followed. Decisions were made on a consensus basis, with the senior staff carrying somewhat more weight. A data sheet (Staff Meeting Rating Form) based on the regular form of the discussions on each patient was used to record the ratings. Interrater reliability and refinement of the instrument were established by a series of trial runs.

In order to explore the hypothesis that there was a patterning of residents' activity with an internal consistency of its own regardless of conference leader, 10 variables which had good interrater reliability and significance were selected from the rating form. A Spearman Rank Order matrix (table) was generated to investigate the relationship of these variables.

On the basis of clinical judgment the investigators noted two major behavior clusters that appeared to be meaningful for purposes of investigation. One cluster had to do with positive perception (seeing one's patient as "improved") and resident's activity; the other with negative perception ("no change" in patient is reported) and resident's activity.

It was found that the resident who reported his patient as being improved was likely to make many requests for his patient; to have many changes agreed on by staff for his patient; to express a positive attitude toward his patient; and to be assertive in his mode of handling the complex interplay of the conference.

It was also found that Staff Caution was correlated with Resident's Requests, Assertiveness, and a positive Therapist's Attitude but was not correlated with the report of patient improvement. Staff Caution referred in this conference to cautioning statements from any member of the staff. It was somewhat less of a "brake" on the resident's autonomous activity than a refusal to grant requests. Clinically it appeared to the observers that if a resident's report about a patient indicated positive attitude and a request for positive change, yet did not follow through with a statement of improvement, the resident

Results of Spearman Rank Order Matrix

	Resident's Requests	Staff Requests	Total Changes	Initiative for Change	Assertiveness	Caution	Therapist's Attitude	Slightly Improved	No Change	Slightly Worse	Tension Level	Tension Indicators
Resident's requests	—	0.33	0.95*	−0.12	0.88*	0.69†	0.90*	0.86*	−0.76†	−0.60	−0.05	−0.43
Staff requests		—	0.33	0.02	0.26	0.67†	0.52	0.17	0.48	−0.47	0.07	−0.88*
Total changes			—	−0.12	0.83*	0.55	0.86*	0.95*	−0.60	−0.55	0.21	−0.33
Initiative for change				—	−0.33	−0.40	−0.21	−0.26	0.04	0.50	−0.40	−0.21
Assertiveness					—	0.74†	0.83*	0.83*	−0.55	−0.45	−0.02	−0.21
Caution						—	0.81†	0.43	−0.74†	−0.71†	−0.19	−0.67†
Therapist's attitude							—	0.79†	−0.64†	−0.62	−0.11	−0.60
Slightly improved								—	−0.36	−0.43	+0.40	−0.11
No change									—	0.74†	0.43	0.67†
Slightly worse										—	−0.12	0.57
Tension level											—	0.24
Tension indicators												—

*$P < 0.01$.
†$P < 0.05$.

was more likely to be seen by the senior staff as being overly optimistic and therefore to be cautioned.

It was quite understandable that improvement should be correlated with the resident's request for privileges. If his patient was unchanged (or "slightly worse"), he was less likely to make requests. A patient who was not doing well might elicit a request for increased medication or restriction. But there was a whole roster of requests that could be called on for a patient making progress; that is, he could be moved to a more advanced group, be given weekend privileges, allowed to eat in the dining room rather than in his room, allowed increased use of hospital facilities, and so on.

It was also the observer's clinical impression that it was when a resident could operate with a high degree of autonomy within the guidelines set down by the hospital that he functioned effectively within this particular milieu. However, a tendency to elicit cautioning statements, despite other positive indications and in the absence of seeing patients as "improved," was an indication that there was a swing in balance from resident autonomy to staff direction. Reporting of patient improvement by the resident was the pivotal factor.

It was found that the resident who reported that his patient showed "no change" was likely to make few requests for his patient. The trend was to have few changes agreed upon by staff for his patient and for the resident to lack assertiveness in handling the interplay of the conference. "No change" was also correlated with a negative attitude toward the patient. Thus there was a similar grouping to that described for seeing one's patient as "improved" only on the negative side. "No change" in the format of this conference implied a rather closed statement which elicited little comment and precluded any real need for making requests.

There was an inverse relationship between Staff Requests and Tension Indicators, as well as between Staff Caution and Tension Indicators. Tension Indicators were all taken together as one group. They reflected the resident's reporting of outside factors as contributing to his difficulty in handling his patient. The trend was that the more positive the attitude expressed toward the patient, the less tendency to mention outside factors

(Tension Indicators) as causing difficulty. In other words, positive patterning appeared to deal with a direct involvement with the patient's status in relationship to the therapist. When the resident expressed the fact that he was having difficulty with the patient arising from seemingly outside factors, there were fewer cautioning remarks by the staff and fewer requests made by them. One could speculate that this indicated that when the resident felt outside pressure, the staff expressed support by not making too many requests or expressing caution. However, this also could have been a reflection of the success of negative defense maneuvers on the part of the resident. That is, by saying that he was having difficulty with his patient due to outside sources, that a referring doctor was causing him difficulty or that the family was interfering, and so forth, he held off possible active intervention by the staff. Thus, so to speak, he provided himself with "an excuse" by projecting difficulties onto outside factors. Such a possibility might only be resolved by more careful study but it was the observer's impression that the latter reasoning fitted the situation better and was a way for the resident to say—"It's their fault, not mine."

Related to this was the fact that Staff Caution was not expressed when there was "no change" reported by the therapist in the patient's condition. Again, since a report of "no change" was one possible approach to handling the conference by shutting out further interaction and discussion, it was understandable that it also eliminated expression of caution. Literally there was nothing to talk about.

It is of interest that the one thing the observers had originally been looking for—the tension level residue of the staff conference—showed no relationship to any of the other categories listed in the data sheet. Actually, it had been hoped that as the observers checked the data sheet they would be able to arrive at an "objective" evaluation of the residual tension from the interaction. What was found instead, and perhaps most interestingly, is that one could not reliably make such "objective" observations. Actual noting of behavioral events was obviously easier than drawing inferences. It was a much more complex and difficult matter to infer and rate the complicated state of "tension." The reliability between the two observers in making this judgment was, as compared with other variables, relatively poor.

CONCLUSIONS

This is, in essence, a pilot study based on a relatively small sampling. It indicates that in this hospital it was possible to identify a patterning of the resident's behavior at the staff meetings which seemed to be consistent over a long span of time. The statistical study yielded a number of significantly related variables in which two major behavior clusters around positive or negative perception of the patient by the reporting therapist and his activity at the staff meeting appear to be particularly meaningful. One cluster had to do with positive perception (seeing one's patient as "improved") and the related variables of positive attitude; making many requests for a patient which were subsequently agreed on by staff; and being assertive. The other had to do with negative perception ("no change" in patient is reported) and the related variables of negative attitude; making few requests for a patient, lacking assertiveness; and mentioning outside or external factors as causing difficulty in the treatment of the patient. Further explorations with larger samples could possibly yield a better understanding of such patterns.

Caudill[2(p337)] in a related search, indicated that residents who were more active at staff meetings were most likely to be rated as superior by their supervisors. This type of correlation was not investigated here, but it was evident that activity was valued in this hospital's staff meetings. There were, however, other specifics which had to be combined with the activity before the resident could gain the assent of the rest of the staff required to carry out his program for a patient.

A central issue at these staff conferences was the negotiations for patient changes and privileges. Success or failure in achieving these might well have a significant effect on the course of individual therapy in the hospital in terms of the residue of attitudes and feelings brought back by the resident. A study of these influences on the therapy hour might help in clarifying some of the complex of interrelationships in this type of institution.

Daniel Zawel performed the statistical consultation and subsequent analyses.

REFERENCES

1. Stanton, A. H., and M. S. Schwartz. *The mental hospital.* New York: Basic Books, 1954.
2. Caudill, W. *The psychiatric hospital as a small society.* Cambridge, Mass.: Harvard Univ. Press, 1958.
3. Etzione, A. "Interpersonal and structural factors in the study of mental hospitals." *Psychiatry,* 23:13–22 (1960).
4. Gralnick, A. "The psychiatric hospital as a therapeutic instrument." In *Collected papers of High Point Hospital,* ed. A. Gralnick. New York: Brunner-Mazel, 1969.
5. Schacht, L. S., and M. Blacker. "Leadership effect on the staff conference process. *Archives of General Psychiatry,* 20:358–64 (1969).

Chapter 18

Therapists' Attitudes and Patients' Clinical Status: A Study of 100 Psychotherapy Pairs

in collaboration with the senior authors, Edwin L. Rabiner, M.D., Morton F. Reiser, M.D., and Harriet L. Barr, Ph.D.

Although definitive studies are long overdue, it is not yet possible to design investigations that could convincingly demonstrate or compare the effectiveness of particular forms of psychotherapy. One major obstacle confronting such research is the lack of a methodology which would adequately take into account the confounding influence of the personal interaction between therapist and patient. Until we are able to define, measure, and control for those characteristics and developments in this highly complex feedback-escalation system which may enhance, impede, or even reverse the effects of the treatment technique being evaluated, the meaning of observed outcomes will be obscure. Favorable outcomes may be as readily attributable to unspecified interactional factors as to the treatment approach itself. Unfavorable outcomes may be similarly inconclusive, in that they may reflect the washing out of positive responses to specified technical operations by negative responses to particular kinds of personal interplay between therapist and patient.

The extent to which situational factors can be expected to influence treatment outcome will obviously depend on the specificity and potency of the treatment agent employed. Thus the emotional climate in which diseased tissue is surgically removed or biochemical mediators of physiological processes are added, neutralized, or removed may be of relatively little consequence. It has been demonstrated, however, that even with treatment agents having a higher order of specificity than psychotherapy can reasonably claim for itself, situational factors can vitiate treatment effectiveness. Two complementary studies on the treatment of essential hypertension speak compellingly to this point. Reiser,[1] using cues obtained in regular debriefing interviews with internists after their treatment contacts with hypertensive patients, reported successfully predicting the occurrence of hypertensive crises on the basis of unconscious hostile attitudes which the patient evoked in the internist during his administration of traditional hypertensive treatment regimens. With apparent implications as to the mediation of these catastrophic sequels, Shapiro[2] noted that hypertensive subjects whose blood pressures dropped in response to alkavervir (Veriloid) when the doctor's attitude was one of enthusiastic commitment, had blood pressure increments when the same drug was given after the doctor's attitude had shifted to one of disinterest and annoyance as a result of distressing developments in the doctor's personal life. The far greater intensity of contact and involvement between the psychotherapist and his patient would appear to maximize the opportunity for such inadvertent negative attitudes in the psychotherapist to similarly influence his patient's response to a treatment approach which might otherwise be effective.

Despite the relative sparsity of investigations attempting to deal intimately with the role of the therapist-patient interaction in the psychotherapeutic process, a measure of empirical support does exist for the notion that psychotherapy can actually be for better or for worse as a consequence of the personal interplay between therapist and patient.

In this regard, Truax[3] found that high levels of such therapist-offered conditions as warmth, accurate, empathic understanding, and genuineness were associated with overall patient improvement, while low levels were associated with patient deterioration. He concluded that, when all therapy was indiscriminately compared to control conditions, there was little average change.

Snyder,[4] using an ongoing self-inventory method; Strupp,[5] using retrospectively completed questionnaires; and Alexander,[6] on the basis of ongoing, intensive, direct observation, have all been led to similar conclusions as to the primacy of the quality of the therapeutic relationship in predicting the success or failure of psychotherapy encounters. As the focal point through which all other psychotherapy variables appear to operate, psychotherapy outcome studies must carefully take into account the character and vicissitudes of the therapeutic relationship. Their failure to do so may be likened to studying the effectiveness of fire extinguishers without bothering to note whether they contain carbon dioxide-producing ingredients or gasoline.

THE PRESENT INVESTIGATION

While it has long been suspected that a psychotherapist's feelings and attitudes toward a given patient both affect and are affected by the patient's clinical state and his responsiveness to the therapist's efforts, the interrelationship between these parameters has not been empirically documented by extensive, systematic observation of sizeable treatment pair samples. The present investigation was designed to provide concurrent data on (1) a broad range of indicators presumed to tap therapists' feelings toward and judgments about their patients, and (2) patients' independently judged clinical status. Its major aim was to identify on an ad hoc basis those dimensions of a psychotherapist's attitudinal set toward a patient which are most intimately linked to the patient's clinical course. Toward this end, a broad spectrum of therapist attitudinal cues was examined in order to determine which cues tended to vary in unison with each other and with patient clinical status over the course of the psychotherapy encounter. The statistical analysis of the obtained data was designed to provide estimates of the extent of mutual interdependence of therapist attitudinal sets toward patients and patient's clinical status; that is, how much the variance in one was accompanied by changes in the other.

It was further hoped that our findings might provide a basis

for constructing an operationally useful self-inventory procedure, by means of which a psychotherapist could, unobtrusively
and on his own, organize his subjective responses to a given
patient along scoring axes reflecting salient aspects of his attitudinal set toward that patient. This would enable therapists themselves to provide uniform, researchable data for use in further
investigations into the role of the therapist-patient interaction in
psychotherapy.

One hundred psychotherapy pairs, meeting for three 45-
minute interviews each week and comprised of psychiatric inpatients and psychiatrists beyond the residency training level,
were monitored on an ongoing basis over periods ranging from
3 to 20 months. Quantitative data on therapists' perceptions
of and feelings toward their patients was provided at biweekly
intervals by the subject therapists and their psychotherapy
supervisors. Concurrent ratings by a well-trained psychiatric
nurse on the ward activity section of the Multidimensional Scale
for Rating Psychiatric Patients (MSRPP) were employed as independent measures of patient's clinical status.[7]

Correlational and factor analytic techniques were used to
determine which among the spectrum of monitored therapist
attitudinal cues tended to vary together over the course of
treatment, thus tapping a common construct, presumably a
salient dimension of the therapist's affective-attitudinal set. The
resulting empirically derived measures were then employed to
examine the extensive data obtained for evidence that how a
therapist feels toward a patient and how the patient is doing
clinically tend to go hand in hand; that is, that shifts in the
psychotherapist's set toward the patient correspond in time and
direction with shifts in the patient's clinical status.

It would obviously have been desirable that the data thus
obtained permit conclusions to be drawn regarding the nature of
the linkage between the therapist's attitudes and the patient's
clinical state; that is, to what extent do therapist attitudes act
upon and to what extent are they acted upon by the patient's
clinical state? This, however, would have required detailed
information about each treatment contact so that it would be
apparent which parameter changed first. The burden of obtain-
ing data on so intensive a basis could have been shouldered only

by the subject therapists if the number of patients rated were substantially reduced. In the present study, priority was given instead to documenting the interdependence of these parameters on an extensive sample containing all the treatment cases of the subject therapists. We would also have had to supplement therapist self-reports of their attitudes toward patients with information about the extent to which these attitudes were objectively manifested and perceived by their patients. The major consideration leading us to forego collection of this data was the likelihood that the direct observational and/or patient self-report procedures required might seriously contaminate the treatment relationships under study. A further consideration was that, in a procedure for measuring therapists' sets toward patients, the inclusion of items requiring outside observers or active patient collaboration would clearly restrict its general usefulness as a research or clinical tool. While they by no means represent adequate substitutes, we did systematically collect the independent observations of psychotherapy supervisors concerning the attitudes which therapists displayed toward their patients during weekly supervisory sessions, along with nurses' ratings of patients' apparent emotional responses to each treatment interview and their overheard comments about their therapists between interviews.

An additional limitation of this work stems from sampling restrictions implicit in the clinical setting in which it was performed. The study sample consisted entirely of hospitalized patients, the bulk of whom carried schizophrenic diagnoses. Moreover, the high cost of private hospital care served to exclude lower status patients from the sample. Furthermore, few assertions can be made as to the representativeness of the nine therapists who participated in the study, other than that they were all beyond the residency training level and viewed themselves as practicing psychoanalytically oriented psychotherapy.

On the other hand, the assignment of patients to therapists on a rotating basis by the hospital's clinical director and the inclusion of the hospital's entire population of psychotherapy pairs during the 20-month study period precluded the operation of a priori or initial preferences on the part of therapists and patients for working together, as well as biases inherent in treatment pair samples comprised of "volunteers" to participate in psychotherapy research.

The major strengths of this study lie in the number of therapy pairs on which its findings are based, its continuous sampling of therapist-patient interactions over extended treatment periods, and its use of an independent observer to provide detailed "objective" judgments of patients' clinical status.

STUDY SAMPLE

Study Setting

This study was performed at High Point Hospital, a private 45-bed psychoanalytically oriented residential treatment center. Its patients are routinely seen for three 45-minute psychotherapeutic interviews a week, regardless of what other treatment adjuvants, including drugs and electroshock, are employed. The treatment program emphasizes therapeutic community concepts, and the major focus of individual psychotherapy is on interpreting the ongoing, inhospital social experience of the patient as he moves through a range of carefully structured and closely observed social interactions in relation to which salient patterns of self-defeat emerge. The hospital's small size provides a relatively homogeneous milieu and permits all administrative and supervisory personnel to become intimately acquainted with all the patients and to participate in all management decisions made for them. (For a more complete description of the treatment ethos, interested readers may refer to a volume of the *Collected Papers of High Point Hospital.*[8])

Subject Sample

During the 20-month period commencing April 1, 1964, the case loads of all psychotherapists at High Point were monitored in the manner described above. One or more biweekly ratings were obtained on all 187 psychotherapy relationships of the nine therapists staffing the hospital during this 20-month period. One hundred fifty-two of these, involving patients admitted after the study began, were monitored from the point of initial therapist-patient contact until either the patient or the therapist left the hospital. Thirty-five of these pairs involved patients already in residence at the hospital. For this group, whose treatment relationships had been established for varying intervals, data was available only for the psychotherapy segments which extended into the study period.

Inasmuch as we were interested in observing the interrelationships among therapist attitudinal and clinical course measures for any and all time segments of a given treatment relationship, no attempt was made to partial-out or balance the sample for this factor.

It should be noted, however, that while initial and later treatment segments are included, pairs comprised of patients leaving the hospital prior to three months of treatment by one therapist were excluded by our lower limit selection criterion. Since the majority of these short-stay patients sign out against medical advice and may be viewed, therefore, as failures with respect to psychotherapeutic engagement, they clearly merit special study. Nevertheless, they were excluded from this investigation because of our wish to base our conclusions on pairs on which data was most extensive. However, a comparison of the 100-pair study sample with the larger group from which it was drawn failed to reveal any significant differences with respect to age, sex, marital status, education, prior hospitalization, or diagnosis.

These 187 relationships were then ordered with respect to the number of consecutive biweekly ratings available for each, and the 100 on whom our data was most extensive were selected as the study sample. The number of rated biweekly treatment segments for these 100 psychotherapy relationships ranged from 6 to 40. The lower limit of 6, which corresponded to 3 months of monitored therapist-patient interaction, seemed to represent an adequate period for relationships to develop definable characteristics and for shifts in these to manifest themselves.

The 100 psychotherapy relationships comprising the study sample involved 9 therapists and 92 different patients. The treatment relationships of seven patients with each of two therapists, and of one patient with each of three therapists, were included. No therapist was represented less than five, nor more than 13, times in the sample.

Clearly, then, while the study sample consisted of 100 different psychotherapy relationships, these were not, strictly speaking, independent of each other. This fact gave rise to uncertainty as to whether the subject sample could be legitimately considered to consist of 100 distinguishable pairs or nine therapists with a total of 100 replications. This uncertainty was resolved by analyses, described later, which revealed marked heterogeneity in the pattern of intercorrelated variables among the treatment pairs contributed by each therapist.

Patients.   There were 32 males and 60 females in the subject group. Ages ranged from 14 to 78, with a mean patient age of 30.9 years and a median age of 27 years. Fifty-eight percent of the patients were less than 30 years old, while patients over 50 years of age represented only 15 percent of the subject sample. There were 43 single, 40 married, 6 divorced, and 3 widowed patients. Fifty-three had attended college, 15 had completed high school, 19 had attended high school, and 5 had not progressed beyond the primary school level. Forty-one patients were undergoing their first psychiatric hospitalization. Seventy-five percent carried schizophrenic diagnoses, with more than one-third being given diagnoses of paranoid schizophrenia. The nosologic distribution of this sample is given in Table 1.

It should be noted, however, that the criteria for diagnosing schizophrenia at High Point Hospital are somewhat broader than those used in many places. Where a patients' social judgment is sufficiently impaired and his life style is sufficiently bizarre, the diagnosis of schizophrenia is made even in the absence of frank secondary symptoms or manifest formal thought disorder. In general, the hospital tends to exclude severely disturbed, regressed psychotics. Thus, while the bulk of the hospital's patient population carries schizophrenic diagnoses, patients tend to be far more intact than state hospital populations and have, for the most part, previously been in psychotherapy with private psychiatrists. It is not uncommon at High Point for patients who were considered by their referring psychiatrists to

Table 1. Nosologic Classification
of Patient Sample

Schizophrenic (N = 69)	
Acute undifferentiated	7
Chronic undifferentiated	18
Paranoid	34
Catatonic	5
Hebephrenic	2
Simple	1
Schizo-affective	2
Psychosis	
Involutional depression	2
Psychotic depression	1
Character disorder	8
Schizoid—Psychopath	2
Psychoneurosis (N = 6)	
Anxiety reaction	2
Reactive depression	2
Mixed psychoneurosis	2
Personality Disorder	
Adjustment reaction of adolescence	3
Chronic brain syndrome	1
Total	92

be in adolescent turmoil or to have severe narcissistic character disorders to be considered schizophrenic.

Therapists. The nine therapists included in the study sample were male. Their ages ranged from 30 to 41, with a mean of 33 years. All therapists had previously completed three years of residency training in psychiatry; the mean prior psychiatric experience for the group was 3.7 years. None were psychoanalytically trained, although three of the group subsequently entered formal psychoanalytic training. The therapists were paid a modest stipend for completing the self-report inventories.

INSTRUMENTS

Guided by a review of the relevant literature and a related prior study we had done on therapists' clinical records,[9] a list of indicators or therapists' affective-additudinal responses to individual patients was compiled. Those items obtainable only through direct observation of treatment interviews, active collaboration of the subject patients, or direct interview of the participating therapists were eliminated. The remaining items were assigned to one of three informant pools (therapist self-report, psychotherapy supervisor, nurse observer) according to which informant had the most ready access to the requisite information. The items in each pool were then scaled and the scales used to construct the rating instruments employed to monitor therapists' emotional sets toward their patients.

Because of the study's heavy reliance on the therapists' self-reports, pains were taken to minimize and circumvent anticipated therapist defensiveness in exposing their feelings about their patients. First, the therapists were assured that the information they provided would be treated as confidential and would not be accessible to the hospital's clinical-administrative staff. Efforts were made in the design of the rating instruments themselves to avoid direct questions as to how the therapist was feeling about a given patient. Inquiries relevant to many evoked feelings and attitudes were couched in terms of patient characteristics rather than the therapists' feelings, on the ground that therapists would be less apt to respond defensively to; "This is the kind of patient who is seductive, sarcastic, clinging, etc." than they would to, "I find myself feeling attracted to, angry at, or rejecting of this patient." With respect to those personal feelings which did not lend themselves readily to this "objectification" strategy, the therapists were asked to rank order all patients in their case loads, thereby forcing discriminations that might otherwise not be made. In these instances, the therapists were also asked to identify the positive, neutral, and negative zones of these rankings, in order to provide for the possibility that a patient might be ranked first, not because he was liked or considered an excellent psychotherapeutic prospect, but because he was less disliked or a better prospect than others with whom the rank orderings compared him.

Therapist Attitude Self-Inventory

This instrument consisted of three major sections. A 23-item "patient characteristic" checklist required the therapists to rate on four-point, intensity-pervasiveness scales the degree to which they perceived their patients as: (1) having an adequate intellectual capacity to engage in insight psychotherapy, (2) ingratiating, (3) denying illness, (4) able to ask realistically for help, (5) sarcastic, (6) hopeless, (7) accepting of therapeutic leadership, (8) openly hostile, (9) able to make valid self-observations, (10) patronizing, (11) maintaining an interesting flow of conversation, (12) nihilistic, (13) manipulative, (14) smiling and pleasant, (15) clinging, (16) appreciating your efforts, (17) negativistic, (18) controlling, (19) hopeful, (20) pleading, (21) seductive, (22) excessively demanding, (23) other (specify).

An eight-item "patient response to treatment" checklist required the therapist to rate (1) the patient's cooperativeness with hospital personnel; the extent to which the patient displayed hostile attitudes toward (2) psychiatry, (3) the hospital, and (4) the therapist, himself; (5) the apparent impact of psychotherapy interviews on the patient's mood and anxiety level; (6) the patient's response to the therapist's efforts to be supportive; (7) the adequacy of the patient's overall progress, and (8) the therapist's level of agreement with other staff members as to how the patient should be managed.

A five-item "subjective reaction" section required the therapists to rank order their case loads and identify the positive, neutral, and negative zones with respect to their (1) overall feelings of liking or disliking the patient, (2) assessment of the patient's psychotherapeutic prospects, (3) level of interest in working with the patient (clock-watching versus where did the hour go?), (4) level of personal comfort versus discomfort during interviews with the patient, and (5) tendency to think about the patient between interviews. Therapists were also asked to indicate those patients who had appeared in any of their dreams during the rating interval. This self-inventory was completed at biweekly intervals by all therapists in relation to all patients in their case loads. Rankings were converted to normalized percentages to equilibrate rank scores given in relation to differing numbers of patients in therapists' case loads at any given time.

Supervisory Ratings of Therapist's Manifest Attitudes

On the basis of weekly supervisory hours in which the subject therapists discussed each of their patients as part of the hospital's ongoing clinical program, psychotherapy supervisors were asked to rate the therapists' attitudes toward their patients. The rating form used provided the following information: (1) the ordinal position in which patients were discussed by their therapists and the length of time devoted to each (including instances in which the supervisor had to remind a therapist that he had not yet discussed a given case); (2) the therapist's apparent affective response to his patient (rated as strongly positive, clinical, objective, indifferent, strongly negative, or indeterminate); (3) the level of goal congruence or therapeutic alliance (rated as excellent, satisfactory, or poor), and, (4) the level of tension in the relationship and the contributions of each participant to it (rated on six-point scales from minimal to maximal). In addition, affect-laden comments about patients, reports of dreams about them, etc., were noted descriptively. These ratings were made each week and averaged to generate biweekly scores.

Nurse Ratings of Patient's Responses to Therapist

The decision made by the investigators to keep patients blind to the research limited the study to essentially two sources of sequential data on patients' feelings toward their therapists: (1) spontaneous comments made to staff members or other patients and overheard by the nursing personnel, and (2) inferences drawn from observations of patient mood and attitude before and after therapeutic interviews. Spontaneous comments about therapists were rated by nursing staff as: *(a)* strongly positive, *(b)* seems satisfied, *(c)* indifferent, *(d)* skeptical-critical, *(e)* strongly hostile, and *(f)* no comments made. Response to sessions was rated as: *(a)* elated, *(b)* in better spirits, *(c)* no apparent change, *(d)* more preoccupied, *(e)* obviously upset, and *(f)* openly hostile to the therapist. The nurses were instructed to record this information in coded form when no patients were present and the data was collected at the end of each nursing tour. At High Point Hospital, sicker patients are accompanied by nursing personnel to and from sessions. More intact patients leave and return on their own to a supervised activity and, therefore, also fall under trained observer scrutiny. Biweekly scores were obtained by averaging the daily ratings. As far as we know, during the 20-month data-collection period no patient became aware that these observations were made.

Clinical Status Measures

Concurrent biweekly assessments of each patient's clinical status were made in the following manner: 42 items were selected on the basis of applicability to the hospital's population from the Lorr Multidimensional Scale for Rating Psychiatric Patients (MSRPP).[7] Only those items which could be completed on the basis of ward observation and which did not require formal interview were chosen. One nurse with a Master's degree in psychiatric nursing completed this inventory biweekly on each patient throughout the study period. In addition, this nurse made a global judgment of clinical change over the biweekly rating interval on a five-point improvement-regression scale. The clinical director and staff meeting observers also rated patients on this scale.

The nurse rater also supplied basic patient data as to which ward the patient was on (open or closed), which activity group (graded I–IV on the basis of increasing demand levels for integrated functioning); drugs administered and dosage levels; electroshock therapy if administered; level of socialization (rated as withdrawn-isolated, passive but responsive, occasionally takes initiative, friendly and outgoing, pushes too hard socially); relationship to personnel (rated as management problem, unpleasant but cooperative, pleasant); number of visits during interval, with whom, where and effect thereof (rated as supportive, anxiety-producing, destructive).

ILLUSTRATIVE PROTOCOL

Before proceeding to the statistical findings constituting the study's hard core, a descriptive summary of the information

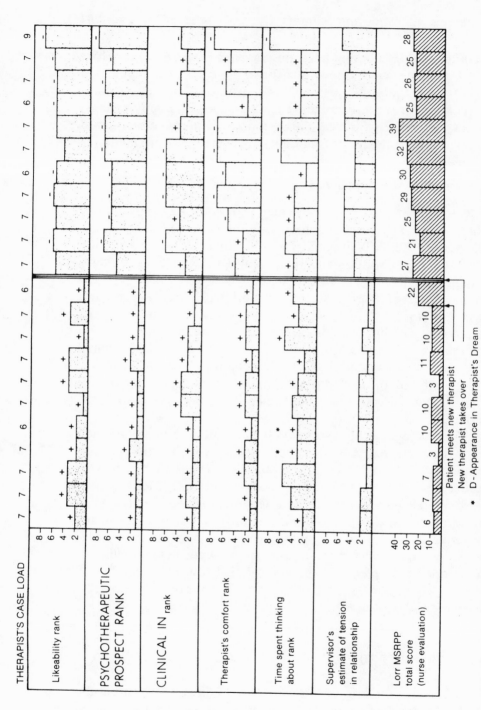

Figure 1. Comparison of a patient's biweekly scores with two successive therapists.

gathered on a single patient with each of two successive therapists is presented and discussed to illustrate the manner in which
our data served to reflect the changing state of affairs between
therapist and patient over the course of their work together.

Figure 1 presents in bar graph form biweekly scores given
patient G.B. on five therapist subjective response measures, one
supervisory measure, and the nurse's MSRPP total score measures during the 3½-month periods preceding and subsequent
to a change of therapist. Bar heights for the upper five measures
indicate the ordinal positions of G.B. in her therapists' case
loads as they vary from interval to interval (that is, the larger the
bar, the more negative the ranking); plus and minus signs indicate whether, apart from her ranked position, G.B. was considered by the therapists to be especially liked or disliked, a particularly good or poor prospect, etc., for the five therapist
subjective response measures. Note that at the point of changeover, all measures reflect a dramatic negative shift; that is, the
second therapist felt far less positively about the patient, he was
judged by his supervisor to have a much stormier relationship to
her, and G.B. appeared considerably sicker to the nurse,
although her clinical retrogression began in the two-week interval when her first therapist was preparing her for the changeover
prior to his departure from the hospital.

Table 2 compares the sums of raw scores on other therapist
self-inventory and nursing measures over the course of the two
time periods. Again, all measures reflect the more negative
attitudinal set of the second therapist toward G.B. This is mirrored in the patient by nurse ratings of her more negative
response to treatment interviews and the dramatic reversal in
the quality of her comments about her therapist, as well as in her
general attitude toward personnel, fellow patients, and the Lorr
measures of clinical status.

As part of the examination of each research protocol, the
ratings given were further compared with whatever collateral
information was available. In the case of G.B., who was treated
by one of us (E.R.) following her hospital discharge, the validity
of the relationship differences depicted in her scores with the
two therapists was clearly confirmed. She had erotic dreams and
fantasies about her first therapist for months after her discharge

Table 2. Comparison of Raw Scores Across 11 Biweekly Rating Intervals

Measure	First Therapist	Second Therapist
Therapist's Patient Characteristic and Response to Treatment Checklist		
Hostile to hospital or therapist	4	10
Impact of sessions: Better	10	6
No change	0	1
Worse	1	5
Responds well to support	32	16
Making adequate progress	29	8
Denies illness	5	15
Asks realistically for help	24	2
Accepts therapeutic leadership	31	13
Makes valid self-observations	26	13
Maintains interesting conversational flow	25	19
Manipulative	18	28
Clinging	15	4
Appreciates therapist's efforts	29	14
Negativistic	4	24
Pleading	2	12
Seductive	21	36
Excessively demanding	3	21
Nursing Observations		
Response to Sessions:		
Number of observations made	69	67
Elated or in better spirits	28	12
Comments overheard	79	56
Rated strongly positive, patient pleased	36	1
Rated strongly negative	1	9
Predominant attitude toward personnel	pleasant, cooperative	management problem
Predominant socialization level	friendly, outgoing	pushes too hard

from the hospital. She described him as warm, sensitive, and intelligent and herself as wanting very much to have him think well of her. In contrast, she described her second therapist as "immature and egotistical" and stated that she had not cared what he thought about her.

Obviously, no conclusions can be drawn as to whether the clinical regression occurring around the change of therapists caused or was caused by the second therapist's negativity toward the patient. It is clear, however, that the kinds of outcome studies done to date, which omit the relationship data presented here, would judge G.B.'s treatment by her second therapist to constitute a clear-cut failure of psychotherapy. Additional data on the prevailing state of affairs between G.B. and her two therapists suggests at the very least, however, that the efficacy of psychotherapy as a treatment method was not clearly tested by her second treatment encounter.

STATISTICAL TREATMENT OF DATA

Analysis of Extreme Changes in Therapist Attitude and Clinical Course

The initial procedure employed in examining the obtained data for evidence that therapist attitudes and patient clinical status are interdependent was to survey those time periods within which the most dramatic changes in either occurred. For this purpose two analyses were performed: the first on only those biweekly intervals characterized by an extreme shift in likeability (112 time periods drawn from 51 therapy pairs) and the second on those periods during which there was an extreme shift in the patient's clinical status as measured by the Lorr Total Score (118 time periods contributed by 43 treatment pairs). While both analyses are referred to in the section on results, only the first of these analyses on extreme likeability change is presented in detail (Table 3) and therefore is used here to illustrate the method employed in both analyses. The criterion for inclusion of a biweekly period in each of these subsamples was that its score change on the particular measure (likeability rank in the first subsample and MSRPP total score in the second) over the two-week period fall within the extreme 5 percent of the distribution of upward or downward shifts for the entire sample of 1,268. Other selected measures taken during each of these time periods were then categorized as changing in the expected or unexpected directions with respect to likeability and clinical status, respectively. For example, if a patient dropped from best-liked to fourth best-liked (a negative therapist attitude shift), while his MSRPP score reflected improvement (a positive

Table 3. Changes in Other Measures During Biweekly Interval When Likeability Rank Changes by 3 or More*

Other Measures	No. Pairs Showing Shift in Same Direction	No. Pairs Showing Shift in Opposite Direction	No. Pairs Showing No Shift	Binomial Probability of Obtained Distribution Occurring by Chance Binominal Expansion $(p + q)^n$
MSRPP total score (Sum of deviations from norm on 42 scales)	32	13	6	0.003
Sum of extent to which patients manifested 8 positive qualities on patient characteristic checklist	36	5	10	0.00001
Sum of extent to which patients manifested 14 negative qualities on patient characteristic checklist	29	8	14	0.00038
Trait balance score (algebraic sum of above two scores)	41	2	8	0.00001
Therapist's statement of like, dislike, or feeling neutral toward patient	38	2	11	0.00001
Psychotherapeutic prospect rank	32	5	14	0.00001
Patient a good, average or poor prospect	18	2	31	0.0002
Clinical interest rank	34	6	11	0.00001
Patient seen as interesting, neutral, or uninteresting	18	4	29	0.002
Comfort level rank	38	8	5	0.00005
Therapist feels comfortable, neutral, or uncomfortable with patient	17	2	32	0.0004
Carry over rank	19	14	18	0.243
Patient given much, average, or little thought	10	10	31	0.59

*Average case load, seven patients. N = 51 doctor-patient pairs over 112 ratings.

clinical status shift), the latter change was considered to be in the unexpected direction. In those instances when a single treatment pair contributed more than one such extreme change time period, the predominant shift pattern among the measures for that pair was determined so that each pair was represented only once in the statistical analyses performed on each extreme change subsample. Sign tests were then used to determine whether when patients clearly became better or less liked by their therapists or markedly improved or regressed clinically, the frequency with which other measures shifted in the expected direction significantly exceeded chance occurrence. The results of these analyses are described below in the section on therapist attitudes and clinical status during periods of dramatic change in one or the other (Table 3).

Data Reduction

As a second step, in order to systematically reduce the 146 biweekly scores obtained by each psychotherapy pair with a minimal loss of information, and in keeping with our interest in organizing the indicators of therapists' subjective responses to a given patient along a smaller number of dimensions representing salient aspects of his emotional set, the following procedure was used. One rating interval was selected on a random basis from those available for each pair in order to insure the inclusion of time samples from all stages of the psychotherapy encounter. Item scores were intercorrelated and the resultant product-moment correlation matrix was factor-analyzed. (Centroid extraction with orthogonal varimax rotation of the eight factors extracted. It should be noted that a matrix in which the variables outnumber the cases is not, strictly speaking, proper. However, since the eight factors obtained were merely used as a guide for the formation of 14 clusters and our purpose was merely to reduce the number of variables, this was not considered a serious problem.) This process helped determine which measures showed little commonality, suggesting their retention as single variables, and which might be combined into empirically and clinically meaningful clusters providing strong and unduplicated measures. Items with low variance were dropped as unsuitable for a correlational study. For those items representing alternative versions or duplications of others, additional tests were run to determine which was the better form.

Twenty-four measures utilizing 65 of the items were thus either derived or selected as those most relevant and presumably useful for the analysis of therapist attitudes and patient status as they vary over time. These are described below.

Therapist Attitude Assessments (Self-Report)

Affirmation of Therapist's Competence Cluster: T_1 (sum of scores on four scales; mean r = 0.67). Consists of the extent to which the therapist judges the patient to: (1) feel better as a result of their talks together, (2) accept his therapeutic leadership, (3) appreciate his efforts and (4) be making adequate overall progress. As such, it appears to tap the degree to which the therapist sees the patient as affirming his professional competence.

Acceptance of Patient Role Cluster: T_2 (sum of scores of four scales; mean r = 0.65). Consists of the extent to which the therapist perceives the patient as able to: (1) ask realistically for help, (2) make valid self-observations, (3) produce interesting material, and (4) respond positively to his efforts to be supportive. While some individual item overlap may exist with T_1, taken as a group these items appear to reflect the patient's manifest acceptance of the psychotherapeutic contract.

Attractive Psychotherapy Patient Cluster: T_3 (sum of normalized percentage scores for three ranked dimensions; mean r = 0.72). Consists of the patient's rank in the therapist's case load with respect to how (1) interesting, (2) comfortable to work with, and (3) promising he is as a psychotherapeutic prospect. It therefore appears to reflect the level of therapeutic gusto he evokes in the therapist.

Provocative Behavior Cluster: T_4 (sum of scores on six scales; mean r = 0.54). Consists of whether, and to what degree the following six presumably irritating behaviors are directed by the patient toward the therapist: sarcasm, open hostility, manipulativeness, negativism, controlling and excessively demanding behavior.

Therapist Liking of Patient: T_5 (one rank order score). The patient's ranking in the therapist's case load with respect to overall personal likeability (as distinct from his role qualities as a patient).

Time Spent Thinking About Patient: T_6 (one rank order score). The patient's ranking in the therapist's case load with respect to the amount of time spent by the therapist thinking about the patient between psychotherapy interviews. Insofar as such carryover may reflect the therapist's involvement with a particular patient, for better or for worse, this single item seemed especially interesting to explore for its correlates with clinical course.

Patient's Hostility Toward the Hospital: T_7—This dichotomous item reflects the occurrence or nonoccurrence of complaining to the therapist about the hospital. As an indirect attack on him, such complaints are apt to generate tension in a hospital therapist. Regardless of the extent to which the therapist may feel identified with the hospital, patient gripes about it require him to defend it or himself, either for choosing to practice there or for having insufficient status to alter its policies.

Therapist's Rating of Patient's Cooperativeness with Hospital Staff: T_8 (score on a single three-point scale). This item attempts to tap the effects of pressures exerted upon the hospital therapist by the social field in which he practices. Complaints by hospital staff members that his patient is a management problem are apt to reflect some degree of covert staff conflict and to arouse concern in the therapist about his professional image.

Supervisory Assessments of Therapist's Attitudes

Relationship Tension Cluster: S_1 (sum of scores on three scales). Comprised of the supervisor's estimate of the level of tension between patient and therapist and the extent to which each participant appears to be contributing to it. It reflects the overall degree of strain or dissonance between therapist and patient as perceived by the supervisor during the therapist's weekly discussion of the patient with him.

Therapist's Enthusiasm Cluster: S_2 (sum of scores on two scales). Comprised of the supervisor's estimates of the extent to which the therapist manifests positive feelings for the patient and clinical interest-enthusiasm for the psychotherapy encounter with him. This judgment was based on the quality of the therapist's affect as he discussed the patient with his supervisor.

Extent of Therapeutic Alliance: S_3 (score on one scale). Supervisory estimate of level of goal congruence between therapist and patient. This assessment reflects the extent to which patient and therapist appear to the supervisor to agree as to the relevance of what is being discussed and done for the patient.

Nursing Staff Assessment

Patient's Response to Sessions: N_1 (score on one 6–point scale). Represents the impact of interviews with the therapist insofar as this was discernible to a nursing staff observer as a mood change in the patient. Scale scores for the six therapy interviews occurring within each biweekly rating period were averaged to obtain a mean session impact score for each rating period.

Patient's Hospital Group Assignment: N_2—At High Point Hospital patients are placed in one of five surveillance-activity groups. Group assignment is made by the medical staff acting in concert on the basis of patient's manifest ability to (1) move about the hospital independently and (2) handle progressively demanding social and task-oriented situations.

Patient's Socialization Level: N_3 (score on one 5–point scale). Represents the overall level from withdrawn-isolated to too socially aggressive at which the patient characteristically socializes with others in the hospital.

Patient's Cooperativeness with Hospital Staff: N_4 (score on one 3–point scale). This is the nursing counterpart of T_8, with which its correlation was 0.27, and represents an overall estimate of the extent to which the nursing staff actually encounters difficulty in managing the patient.

Patient's Overall Clinical Status: N_5 (sum of deviations from healthy behavior on 42 scales of the Ward Activity section of the Lorr MSRPP). This score combines both the extent of psychopathology on single symptom dimensions and the number of dimensions on which the patient deviates. It is thus a measure of the extent of a patient's overall pathology as manifested in his ward activity.

Mood-Activity Level Cluster: N_6 (sum of weighted deviations on seven MSRPP scales mean $r = 0.71$). Lorr's original factor weightings were superseded by those derived from the present analysis. Weights were assigned on the basis of the factor structure generated in the analysis of the 146×146 correlation matrix. This measure reflects the patient's general activity level from inhibited-inactive through manic hyperactive.

Sociability Cluster: N_7 (sum of weighted deviations on four MSRPP scales; mean $4 - 0.65$). Overlaps with N_3 with which it is highly correlated, but is based on specifically defined social interactional characteristics, including number of interests and volubility.

Psychoticism Cluster: N_8 (sum of weighted deviations on eight MSRPP scales; mean $r = 0.62$). The degree to which the patient's gross behavior reflects underlying psychotic thinking (hallucinations, delusions, fragmentation).

Regression Cluster: N_9 (sum of weighted deviations on three MSRPP scales; mean $r = 0.69$). Reflects the extent of

grossly regressed behavior (helplessness, assaultiveness, slov-
enliness).

Somatization Cluster: N_{10} (sum of deviations on two
MSRPP scales; mean = 0.63). Reflects the extent of physical
complaints and bodily concerns.

Belligerence-Resistiveness Cluster: N_{11} (sum of deviations
on six MSRPP scales; mean r = 0.57). Reflects the extent to
which the patient's ward behavior is characterized by resistance, uncooperativeness, irritability, profanity, hostility, and
bullying.

Self-Depreciation Cluster: N_{12} (sum of weighted deviations
on two MSRPP scales; mean r = 0.66). Reflects the degree to
which patient's behavior is self-depreciating and denigrating, as
opposed to conceited and grandiose.

Patient Receiving Electroshock: N_{13}. Scored *yes* if electroshock therapy was administered during the biweekly rating
interval. This item was included solely as a means of testing the
assumption that the prescription of electroshock therapy might
result, as many have suggested, from a negative shift in the
therapist's attitude toward his patient, rather than as a response
to some symptomatic indication.

Interrelationship of Therapist Attitudes and Clinical
Status Within and Across Treatment Pairs

All 1,268 biweekly periods over which data on the sample's
100 therapy pairs had been obtained were then scored on these
24 measures. For each pair, 24×24 product-moment correlation matrices were generated, reflecting the actual intercorrelation
of each variable with the other variables as they fluctuated from
time period to time period over the course of the psychotherapy
encounter.

All 100 matrices were then examined in relation to the patterning of their significant intercorrelations. Four subgroups,
into which 66 of the 100 cases clearly fell, were identified on the

basis of the configurations of significant intercorrelations. The finding that the treatment relationships contributed by each of the nine therapists and 92 different patients were distributed across, rather than confined within subgroups, appeared to warrant the assumption that our sample represented 100 relatively independent subjects rather than nine subjects (the therapists) with a total of 100 replications. Separate factor analyses were done on each of these subgroups, and these will be reported on elsewhere. Suffice it to say in this report that, despite differences in subgroup factor structures, there were sufficient similarities across all four subgroups to warrant their inclusion in a combined factor analysis performed in order to define the data's major trends with respect to which measures were mostly intimately associated over the course of the psychotherapy encounter. This analysis (centroid extraction with oblique rotations) was performed on standardized scores based on their distributions within therapy pairs. Since standard scores express only variations over time, differences across pairs were thus partialled out. The results of this factor analysis on the 66 pairs which typed, are given in Table 4.

It should be noted that when the 66 pairs selected for factor analysis were compared with the remaining 34, they were found to be similar in all major respects. The unused cases differed only with respect to having fewer rating intervals, less clinical status variability and, consequently, fewer significant intercorrelations in their matrices. Because these several aspects of data insufficiency would have diluted the results, these cases were excluded from the factor analysis. Grossly similar, although slightly lower interrelationships among the measures were, indeed, apparent in the mean intercorrelations computed on the full sample of 100.

FINDINGS

Therapist Attitudes and Clinical Status During Periods of Dramatic Change in One or the Other

Table 3 indicates that during biweekly treatment segments when therapist liking of a patient took a decided up or down

Table 4. Oblique Factor Pattern and Structure (N = 918 Rating Intervals Contributed by 66 Classifiable Pairs)

Variable	Variable Description	Loading*	Correlation Between Variable and Factor		
			I	II	III
	Factor I				
	Therapist Attitudinal Set				
T_1	Patient provides little affirmation of therapist's competence	0.75	0.76	0.40	0.34
T_2	Patient poorly accepts patient role	0.72	0.77	0.37	0.48
T_3	Patient viewed as unattractive psychotherapy candidate	0.69	0.63	0.18	0.30
T_5	Therapist feels negatively toward patient	0.60	0.55	0.22	0.21
T_4	Patient exhibits substantial provocative behavior	0.58	0.61	0.45	0.19
S_1	Supervisor judges tension in relationship to be substantial	0.57	0.48	0.10	0.19
S_3	Supervisor judges therapeutic alliance to be poor	0.50	0.42	0.11	0.25
S_2	Supervisor judges therapist to feel negatively toward and disinterested in the patient	0.46	0.40	0.09	0.18
T_8	Therapist presumes patient to be uncooperative with staff	0.37	0.49	0.48	0.23
T_7	Therapist reports patient to be hostile toward hospital	0.35	0.33	0.22	0.05
	Factor II				
	Obtrusive Sick Behaviors				
N_{11}	Belligerent-resistive vs cooperative	0.72	0.10	0.51	−0.08
N_5	Sicker overall clinical status (MSRPP score)	0.67	0.41	0.79	0.62
N_{10}	Tends to have bodily complaints	0.58	0.30	0.60	0.33
N_8	Psychotic thinking	0.57	0.36	0.68	0.53
N_4	Nurse rates patient as uncooperative with staff	0.46	0.37	0.52	0.23
N_9	Regressed behavior	0.41	0.23	0.47	0.36
T_8	Therapist presumes patient to be uncooperative with staff	0.35	0.49	0.48	0.23
	Factor III				
	Unobtrusive Sick Behaviors				
N_6	Depressed-inhibited vs manic-hyperactive	0.74	0.29	0.24	0.68
N_{12}	Self-depreciating vs grandiose	0.71	0.19	0.19	0.61
N_7	Withdrawn (MSRPP sociability cluster)	0.63	0.44	0.59	0.77
N_{11}	Belligerent-resistive vs cooperative	−0.38	−0.10	−0.51	0.08
N_2	In a poorer hospital group	0.38	0.35	0.35	0.49
N_5	Sicker overall clinical status (MSRPP Total Score)	0.35	0.41	0.79	0.62
N_3	Unsociable	0.35	0.41	0.44	0.50

*Only loadings exceeding 0.35 are listed.

swing, the frequencies with which both patient clinical status and other aspects of therapist sets toward patients showed correspondingly positive or negative shifts significantly exceeded chance occurrence. The 13 listed measures were selected or derived or both from the original pool of indicators on the basis of a priori judgments of their presumed saliency. The first four of these are summary scores that combine 64 separate items. Note that the only measures that vary independently of whether the patient is better or less liked deal with the amount of time therapists spend thinking about patients between sessions.

When we examined 118 treatment segments contributed by 43 treatment pairs during which MSRPP total scores shifted 15 or more points up or down (signifying a substantial clinical improvement or regression), the findings similarly confirmed the tendency for therapist attitude indicators to move in the same direction as the patient's clinical status. While clearly discernible trends in five of the last six therapist attitude measures listed in Table 3 failed to reach significance, six therapist attitude measures showed the anticipated distribution of associated shifts at beyond the 0.05 level. Shifts in patients' likeability rank were in the anticipated direction at the 0.006 level.

In order to determine whether the observed tendency for therapist attitudes and clinical status to shift in the same direction might have been mediated by the effects of drugs on both, these analyses were repeated on treatment segments during which there had been no change in patient's medication. Similar levels of associated change among the measures of therapist attitude and patient status during drug constant intervals suggested that their observed interdependence was not attributable to drug effect.

Observed Interrelationship Between Therapist Attitudes and Clinical Status Within and Across Therapy Pairs

Table 4 presents the pattern and structure obtained from the factor analysis of the 918 biweekly ratings contributed by the 66 therapy pairs on which our data was most extensive. The three-factor solution thus obtained defines the principal trends in the data with respect to measures varying in most intimate association with each other. Seven of the eight measures of therapist attitudes employed in the study were placed in factor I, supporting the findings of other investigators[10,11] that psychotherapists' emotional responses to patients (liking, comfort level, interest-enthusiasm, professional role satisfaction) are intertwined with and almost inseparable from their clinical judgments about patients (psychotherapeutic prospects, progress in treatment, etc.). Factors II and III consist essentially of clinical status measures and represent internally consistent, but qualitatively different, aspects of patient's psychopathology. Factor II indicates that obtrusive or outwardly directed sick behaviors (belligerence, complaining, psychotic, regressed behaviors) tend to change in unison, while factor III indicates a similar trend among less obtrusive sick behaviors (depression, self-depreciation, withdrawn, cooperative versus resistant). While the highest level of interrelationship is clearly between measures placed within each of the three obtained factors, the substantial inter-correlations of measures placed in one factor with the other two factors demonstrates that the individual therapists' attitudinal components of factor I are significantly linked to the two constellations of pathological behaviors defined by factors II and III. More significantly, with respect to the major aim of this study, all three of the obtained factors were found to be substantially intercorrelated.

Table 5 indicates that the overall correlation between the therapist's attitudinal set, as defined by factor I, and obtrusive

Table 5. Factor Intercorrelations

	I	II	III
I Therapist attitude		0.49	0.48
II Obtrusive sick behavior			0.48
III Unobtrusive sick behavior			

sick behaviors, as defined by factor II, was 0.49, while the correlation with unobtrusive sick behaviors, as defined by factor III, was 0.48. Thus the levels of therapist's attitudinal sets as measured by factor I are linked to the levels of both kinds of psychopathology. More negative therapist attitudes are associated with sicker patient behaviors. While the direction of this linkage (that is, which is cause and which effect) cannot be established by a correlational study of this kind, there is clearly a substantial interdependence between therapists' attitudes toward and perceptions of a patient and the patient's clinical status, with each accounting for approximately one quarter of the variance in the other. The correlation of 0.48 between factors II and III simply reflects the fact that they measure different, although somewhat related, forms of psychopathology.

Of the 24 measures studied, only three failed to load substantially (> 0.35) on one of the three factors obtained. These appear to be relatively independent of the other measures. The time therapists spend thinking about patients between sessions (T_6) appears, for this sample of therapy pairs, to be quite unrelated to the other attitudinal indicators and clinical measures studied. Conceivably, therapists may think more about both "better" and "poorer" patients. Product-moment correlations could not be expected to pick up any such curvilinear relationship.

The patient's observed response to sessions (N_1), the sole measure tapping, albeit indirectly, the therapist's personal impact on the patient, had only a negligible loading on factor I (0.20), although this was higher than its loadings on the other factors (0.12 and 0.07, respectively). Its apparent independence of the other measures may simply mean that patients' reactions to therapists' attitudes toward them were not discernible to nursing staff raters by the procedure used.

Since only 14 patients received electroshock therapy during the study period, its failure to load adequately on one of the three factors was hardly surprising. For those pairs within which electroshock therapy was administered, the other variables in the analysis did not predict the particular time intervals when it was given. Comparison, however, of the shock group's overall mean attitude and clinical scores (prevailing levels throughout the psychotherapy encounter) with those for the total sample revealed several interesting differences which are worthy of comment. These are presented in Table 6.

While nosological classification failed to discriminate the shock and nonshock groups, mean preshock scores on several

Table 6. Characteristics of Group Receiving Electroshock Therapy*

Differences at 0.01 Level	Differences at 0.05 Level	Differences at 0.10 Level
T_1 Little affirmation of therapist's competence	T_2 Poor acceptance of patient role	S_2 Low therapist enthusiasm
older—median age = 44	(Does not respond well to support,	(Supervisor judges therapist as feeling
(Poor prospect, uninteresting and	cannot ask realistically for help, does	bored and burdened and disliking
tending to make therapist	not make valid self-observations, does	patient.)
uncomfortable.)	not maintain interesting flow of	N_2 In lowest hospital group
N_5 High MSRPP Total Score	conversation.)	N_4 Management problem
N_6 Inhibited—Inactive	N_3 Withdrawn	N_{11} Cooperative rather than belligerent
N_7 Withdrawn	(nurse rating of socialization level)	
N_8 Psychotic thinking	N_9 Regressed	
N_{12} Self-depreciatory	N_{11} Bodily complaints	

*Listed according to probability level (significant levels determined by Chi-square) re-distribution of shock group above and below means of listed variables for 100 therapist-patient pairs.

therapist attitude measures, as well as on the psychopathology components of factor III, were associated with the decision of a therapist to use electroshock therapy. Shock patients were given significantly lower overall ratings with respect to both affirming their therapist's competence and accepting a patient's role. These findings cannot be construed as either clearly supporting or refuting the conjecture of many that the prescription of electroshock therapy is a phenomenon of negative countertransference. The significant intercorrelations of the affirmation of therapists' competence and the acceptance of patient role clusters with factor III (0.34 and 0.45, respectively; see Table 4) suggests that therapists, in fact, are apt to experience their psychotherapeutic endeavors with depressed, self-depreciating, withdrawn patients as unrewarding, so that therapist negativity and the classical symptomatic indications for electroshock therapy may actually represent two sides of the same coin.

Returning now to the measures of therapist attitudes which are found to have the greatest tendency to vary in unison over time, the supervisory assessments do not appear, from their loadings which range from 0.46 to 0.57, to contribute sufficiently to the therapist's attitude factor to warrant the rather cumbersome supervisory procedure they require. While, for purposes of the present study, they provided a measure of concurrent validity, helping to establish the meaning of the underlying construct tapped by factor I, they are not likely to be available in most psychotherapy settings.

The five measures with the highest loadings on the therapist's attitude factor, which are readily available in all psychotherapy settings, are of great interest with respect to their level of association with patient's clinical status. Table 7 lists the means of the within pair correlations of each of these measures with the MSRPP total score (the best overall measure of patient status). For both the entire sample and the 66 pairs included in the factor analysis, all mean correlations were different from zero at well beyond the 0.001 level of significance. The failure among the 34 unused pairs for three of the five mean correlations to reach significance appears, as has already been indicated, accountable to various aspects of data insufficiency.

Table 7. Mean Within Pair Correlations Between MSRPP Total Scores and Five Salient Therapist Attitude Measures*

Measures Correlated	All 100 Pairs (N = 1268 Time periods)		66 High Variance Pairs (N = 918 Time periods)		34 Inadequate Variance Pairs (N = 350 Time periods)	
	Mean†	1% Confidence Limits	Mean	1% Confidence Limits	Mean	P = Value vs 0
Affirmation of therapists competence cluster × MSRPP	0.391	(0.509/0.259)	0.524	(0.641/0.384)	0.099	NS
Acceptance of patient role cluster × MSRPP	0.403	(0.521/0.271)	0.505	(0.633/0.347)	0.189	0.05
Attractive psychotherapy patient cluster × MSRPP	0.309	(0.428/0.180)	0.352	(0.518/0.174)	0.227	0.01
Provocative patient behavior cluster × MSRPP	−0.353	(−0.481/−0.210)	−0.438	(−0.582/−0.267)	−0.170	NS
Therapist liking of patient cluster × MSRPP	0.208	(0.324/0.086)	0.298	(0.417/0.167)	0.034	NS
Affirmation of therapists competence cluster × acceptance of patient role cluster	0.804	(0.864/0.723)	0.831	(0.892/0.738)	0.745	0.001

*Means and standard errors of means on which 1% confidence limits are based were derived by transformation of r in Fisher's z which is normally distributed; the resulting figures were then converted back to r.

†P 0.001 for all means.

COMMENT

Longitudinal study of a large sample of psychotherapy pairs revealed that a number of diverse aspects of psychotherapists' attitudinal responses to their patients vary in intimate relationship to each other over the course of the psychotherapy encounter. These included:

1. The therapists' perception of the extent to which the patient: (a) responded positively and appreciatively to his efforts (T_1); (b) approximated in his interview behavior an "ideal psychotherapy patient" (T_2); (c) behaved considerately in relation to both the therapist (T_4) and the nursing staff (T_8); (d) showed no rancor toward the hospital to whose staff the therapist belonged (T_7).
2. The therapist's feeling of comfort with interest in and therapeutic optimism about the patient (T_3).
3. The therapist's feeling that he liked the patient (T_5).

Apparently, therefore, at times when patients' attitudes and behavior in the dyadic situation are most consistent with therapists' personal and professional interests, providing affirmation of the effectiveness of their "science," their competence in its use, and even of the institution with which they are affiliated, therapists find patients more likeable and savor more their work together. Independent evaluations made by psychotherapy supervisors lent further credence to the interpretation that these covarying facets of a psychotherapist's response to his patient reflect a more generalized, underlying, positive-negative, attitudinal set in the therapist. This set appears closely tied to the level of gratification the patient is providing for the therapist.

This finding is similar to that reported by the Snyders[4] in a study on a more restricted therapy pair sample. They found substantial intercorrelations between a therapist's rankings of clients on dependence, guardedness, rapport, success of therapy, and amount liked by the therapist.

The positiveness-negativeness of therapists' sets toward their patients were further found to be highly related to patients' independently judged clinical status. Thus therapists were more positively disposed toward patients at times when patients appeared less ill to the nurse and more negatively disposed when patients appeared sicker. This finding may be attributable to one or both of two cause and effect sequences. On the one hand, therapists may feel more positively disposed toward patients because they appear to be getting better. On the other, patients may get better because they perceive a more positive attitude toward them in their therapists. Unfortunately, the correlational techniques employed in this study do not permit conclusions to be drawn as to the relative contributions of either causal sequence to the empirically demonstrated interdependence between therapist's attitudes and clinical status.

It is, however, the magnitude of this interdependence which constitutes the major finding of this study. The obtained correlations of 0.48 and 0.49 between the therapist's attitude factor and the two clinical status factors means that each accounts for approximately one quarter of the variance of the other. The positiveness-negativeness of therapist attitudes thus looms as a highly significant variable in the psychotherapeutic process. To the extent that therapeutic change may be an effect of therapists' attitudes, assessments of therapists' attitudes cannot be omitted from meaningful outcome studies. On the other hand, to the extent that therapist expectancies of their work with patients are determined by a patient's clinical status at any given point in treatment as part of a more generalized positive-negative set, their objectivity must be called into question.

Since measures showing little or no change cannot achieve the levels of intercorrelation required for factor analytic clustering, our findings indicate that psychotherapists bear little resemblance to "standardized psychotherapeutic instruments" but, rather, are characterized by considerable variability in their feelings about and perceptions of their patients over the course of the psychotherapy encounter. Insofar as similar attitudinal fluctuations have been noted in therapist samples comprised of senior psychoanalysts[6] and experienced Rogerian therapists,[5] they appear to cut across theoretical persuasions and levels of experience. While differences between therapists (for example, interest patterns,[12] warmth, genuineness, empathy,[3] and expressiveness[13]) have received a measure of attention in the literature, intratherapist differences over the course of a single psychotherapy encounter of the sort revealed in the present investigation have been ignored, for the most part, in research reports. However, it must be conjectured that the magnitude, frequency, duration, and timing of shifts in a therapist's set toward a patient play a significant role in both the efficiency and ultimate outcome of psychotherapy.

The emergence in this study of a single, clearly defined positive-negative therapist-attitude factor has a further practical application. The two therapist-attitude measures which were most highly correlated with this factor and therefore best reflect the level of therapist positiveness were also found to be most highly correlated with the best overall measure of clinical status. These were the acceptance of patient role and the affirmation of therapists' competence clusters. These are conceptually interrelated and together encompass eight 4-point scales which can be completed by a therapist in two or three minutes for each patient he treats. Since these two clusters are highly intercorrelated (0.804, full sample), the use of both does not add appreciably to the MSRPP variance predicted by one. Nevertheless, the use of all eight of their component scales provides a more reliable measure of the construct tapped by the therapist attitude factor. While contributions to this construct are also made by the therapist's feelings toward the patient of liking, being comfortable with, interested in, enthusiastic about the psychotherapeutic prospects of, and being unburdened by high levels of the six provocative patient behaviors measured by T_4, these two clusters appear to reflect adequately the status of the underlying attitudinal dimension. They showed sufficient variability both within and across treatment pairs to discriminate adequately levels at which this attitudinal dimension is present.

Beyond the presumably constructive effects on therapists of the introspection these appraisals require, they appear to be useful as nonobtrusive and readily applicable means of taking into account a basic component of his affective involvement with a patient which, on the basis of this study, is closely tied to the patient's clinical status and, therefore, presumably to treatment outcome.

The variability in therapist attitudes and clinical status which characterized our therapy pair sample has an additional methodological implication. Thorny problems of criterion adequacy and sample attrition are generally encountered in research designs using overall treatment outcome as the dependent variable in relation to which the role of other psychotherapy variables may be investigated. The use of consecutive ratings on multiple measures over relatively brief segments of the total treatment encounter appears to represent a feasible and promising alternative strategy in settings where detailed, independently judged sequential clinical status data is obtainable. The present study demonstrates the usefulness in hypothesis-seeking research on the psychotherapeutic process of such longitudinal studies of individual dyads.

This study was supported in part by grants M 05392 and MH 08018 from the National Institute of Mental Health and by the Gralnick Foundation, Port Chester, N.Y.

REFERENCES

1. Reiser, M. *et al.* "The influence of countertransference attitudes on the course of patients with hypertension in medical treatment." *Journal of American Psychoanal. Association,* 1:566–68 (1953).

2. Shapiro, A. P. *et al.* "Comparison of blood pressure response to veriloid and to the doctor." *Psychosomatic Medicine,* 16:478–87 (1954).

3. Truax, C. "Effective ingredients in psychotherapy: an approach to unraveling the therapist-patient interaction." *Journal of Consulting Psychologists,* 10:256–63 (1963).

4. Snyder, W. U., and B. J. Snyder. *A Psychotherapeutic Relationship.* New York: Macmillan, 1961.

5. Strupp, H. *et al.* "Psychotherapy experience in retrospect." *Psychol. Monographs,* 78:1–45 (1964).

6. Alexander, F. "The dynamics of psychotherapy in the light of learning theory, summarized." *Bulletin of the Phil. Association of Psychoanalysts,* 14:47–49 (1964).

7. Lorr, M. *A multidimensional scale for rating psychiatric patients.* Technical bulletin 10507. Washington, D.C.: Veterans Administration, 1953, 6:1–42.

8. Gralnick, A. *Collected papers of High Point Hospital: the psychiatric hospital as a therapeutic instrument*. New York: Brunner-Mazel, 1969.

9. Rabiner, E. L., and A. Gralnick. "Transference-countertransference phenomena in the choice of shock." *Archives of Neurological Psychiatry*, 81:517–21 (1959).

10. Wallach, M. S., and H. H. Strupp. "Psychotherapists' clinical judgments and attitudes toward patients." *Journal of Consulting Clinical Psychologists*, 24:316–23 (1960).

11. Welkowitz, J. *et al*. "Value system similarity: investigation of patient-therapist dyads." *Journal of Consulting Clinical Psychologists*, 31:48–55 (1967).

12. Betz, B. J. "Studies of the therapist's role in the treatment of the schizophrenic patient." *American Journal of Psychiatry*, 123:963–77 (1967).

13. Rice, L. N. "Therapist's style of participation and case outcome." *Journal of Consulting Clinical Psychologists*, 29:155–60 (1965).

Chapter 19
Treatment Considerations in the Adolescent Inpatient (Report on 92 Cases Compared with 92 Adults)

in collaboration with Edwin L. Rabiner, M.D., Guillermo del Castillo, M.D. and Daniel Zawel, M.S.

When one subjects his ideas and methods to scrutiny—particularly if they are in an area of dispute—a review of several aspects of the program which they constitute would seem in order. These should include (1) the history, (2) the determinants, including those of an extraneous character, which prompted and promoted the program, (3) the experience of the program in operation, (4) the rationale developed to justify its continuation despite contrary methods by equally capable colleagues, and (5) the results with patients, the program's unwitting subjects.

Although every program has its unique qualities, we can clarify the origins and nature of our own by expanding on the above-mentioned aspects. When we started our hospital in 1951 for the treatment of adults, it was commonly accepted that children were treated separately, adolescents in their own "unit," and adults apart from both. We had no idea then that we would do anything contrary. However, one night in that first year a colleague appealed for assistance with an emergency situation. He had in his office a 13-year-old who was acutely disturbed. The patient had been making life miserable for his parents, had been assaulting them, and this very evening had begun to "break up the furniture." Would we admit him? The local institution for adolescents could not take him. Would we

266

"hold the patient for a day or two" until the "proper" admission could be made?

What was our dilemma? We had about 35 open beds! But how could one admit an adolescent into a hospital for adults? And what did we know about his hospital treatment among adults? Could we in good conscience accept him without feeling the profession's criticism of such a step? Would some think we were taking him merely to "fill a bed"? These were some of the questions going through the mind of the admitting physician as he listened to the insistent appeal for help. "Well," he finally said, "I guess there can't be much harm done, but please remember—only for a couple of days." In 30 minutes two tense, distraught, but thankful parents arrived with their slight, sullen son who looked rather pitiful and in sad need of a haircut. He offered no objections to his admission and seemed relieved that he would soon be separated from his parents.

One can guess what happened. The institution for adolescents could not admit him, and the "few days" stretched into some three months. The youngster did wonderfully well. Personnel and other patients rallied about him, and in short order he was at home. His relationship with his parents improved markedly, and he developed a fine working relationship with his therapist. When he finally was transferred he protested, cried bitterly, and pleaded to remain.

Unfortunately, this experience did not prompt us to reach out for adolescents as patients. This was not to our credit, for we did not learn as readily as we should have, nor were we as courageous as we might have been at that time. However, "necessity" on various occasions did require or "permit" us to admit adolescents at a steadily increasing rate. Finally, probably about 12 years ago, it became our conviction, regardless of common practice and thinking on the subject, that adolescents should be by preference admitted into an adult unit. We then actively encouraged their admission, set about formulating and propounding our program for them, and began to see them for the sick people they really are. We found, too, that our rationale for their treatment seemed the same as for older patients and that they responded to essentially the same program provided adults. Subsequently the flood of adolescent admissions arrived for us as it did for all other hospitals, but we were quite prepared for it.

In 1959, 20 percent of our admissions were adolescents. From that point through 1966 our average annual adolescent admission rate was 25.3 percent, compared to 9.4 percent during the preceding eight years. Further, we found ourselves giving an increasing proportion of our time to the daily treatment of adolescents. Thus the percentage of adolescent patient-days between 1959 and 1966 fluctuated from 24 to 51 percent of the total patient-days spent in the hospital, for an average of 35 percent. Accordingly, we could not help but be convinced that a definite change had come upon the psychiatric scene. At the moment it is only with effort that we keep the percentage of adolescents in residence at any one time down to 45 to 55 percent. Our treatment rationale requires us to do so. However, were our thinking different, we could become "a hospital for adolescents" merely by letting the profession know that this was our intention. The demand seems to be that great. Yet no matter how high our percentage of adolescents, we do not feel that we are such a hospital, nor do we seem to experience an uncommon amount of difficulty on that account.

The custom of speaking about "The Adolescent Within an Adult Treatment Program" suggests that the adolescent is out of place in such a program and that he could hardly be treated adequately in it. How then can we characterize the program in which he comprises 40 to 50 percent or more of the patients? Would we title a paper devoted to it, "The Adult Within an Adolescent Treatment Program"? Hardly! Yet we need to think about the matter and recast our thinking. The general population is becoming younger; soon the majority of it will be under 25. Our hospital patient population will reflect these figures and undoubtedly soon will be composed of a majority of adolescents. What then? In this context, we think of High Point Hospital as having a unitary program—one in which similarly sick people of various ages are treated. We scout both the idea that adolescents are shortchanged among adult patients and the thought that adults necessarily suffer adverse effects when exposed to adolescents. They can learn from each other and profit from association under the single roof of a hospital properly organized and oriented. We think of our own program as so designed. How are we to think of the family composed of four adolescents and two parents? Who is living with whom? And which group has priority? In the healthy family a common bond and purpose, more or less accepted by all, will make for harmonious living and positive accomplishment for each. Anything less than this leads to trouble. The implications for the hospital are apparent. We believe our younger patients gain a more sympathetic appreciation for the problems of the older person, including their parents, and that our older patients gain a similar understanding of the younger person, including their own children.

It seems to us that the young person in the purely "adolescent unit" is in a rather artificial atmosphere. In real life he lives with adults and is exposed to the problems he has with them. While it is true that the personnel of a hospital are adults, the contact with them does not have the same impact as does the actual living together with adult patients. The youngster has a common bond, namely, the illness, and shares a similar experience with them. He therefore "accepts" and learns from such sick adults with whom he is in sympathy.

We believe that the problems of adolescents stem primarily from their relationships with adults rather than their peers. Among peers they are more comfortable and find allies to support their sick behavior. Unless counterbalanced, this leads to the unmanageable trouble in the gang and the "hospital for adolescents." It is among adults that the adolescent's difficulties are evoked more easily for study and remedy, rather than merely being "acted out" violently. Accordingly, we tend to deemphasize the importance of the peer group as such and to view the peer group atmosphere as artificial for the hospital. We have groups of patients, not peers, and they are perforce generally mixed in sex as well as age.

In a group program with adults it is easier to define and teach socially acceptable behavior and ultimately a healthy aggression which stems from a rational appraisal of reality. In this context we emphasize productive activity rather than leisure-time recreation. We refer to our young people as patients—not adolescents—as we do to others in any other age group. Each has his role and responsibility, as do all other patients. As with adults, the nature of the therapist's personality has much to do with the end results achieved, as has the age, personality, and basic attitudes of the nursing personnel toward younger people. We accept and respect truly "adolescent" behavior, but will tamper with it when it stems from psychopathology. In this respect we are equally tolerant of behavior characteristic of other age groups.

The hospital staff which treats adolescents is faced with many questions to answer, as well as problems to solve. What age comprises the adolescent group? When is an adolescent no longer such, but instead an "adult"? Is an adult ever "adolescent"? Does the adolescent mainly suffer with a disease process or is "adolescent turmoil" and ego-fragmentation his main difficulty? Are his symptoms evanescent or do they comprise a persistent disease entity which requires diagnosis and treatment? Is "turmoil" natural to all adolescents? If so, how do we distinguish the normal from the disturbed? Need we treat him or merely "support" him until he "grows out of his trouble"? May it be that the disease process itself has caused the ego impairment? This last is a very critical question we must answer for ourselves. If the answer is "yes," then it would seem that the disease must be attacked if rehabilitation is to be possible. Put another way, reversing the disease process may very well be synonymous with reconstitution of the ego!

In any event, how do we go about treating the adolescent if we consider him sick? Should it be psychotherapy, drug therapy, shock therapy, or milieu therapy? Or a combination of them? Do we house him only with his peers or together with adults? Now that he fills so many beds, do we treat him among adults by choice and in keeping with sound principles or because we have no alternative and therefore at the sacrifice of our basic beliefs? If we believe he should be treated among his peers, what are our handicaps and personal problems as therapists when the bed situation denies us our choice? Do we perhaps find ourselves trying to combine a "program for adolescents" and "a program for adults" under the same roof, and come to grief thereby? In other words, does the present limitation of beds permit consistency between our theoretical orientation and our clinical practice? Further, what effect must the presence of adolescents have on the open-door policy of a hospital?

We ourselves believe that the great majority of adolescents hospitalized with us suffer a disease entity, namely schizophrenia, rather than an evanescent symptom picture loosely described as "adolescent turmoil." We believe that most of the "behavior problems" who come to us are psychotic people and that they are sick much earlier in life than we usually suspect. We believe that the adolescent's "rebelliousness" and "problem with authority" are often evidence of his distortion of reality, for example, of paranoid attitudes toward those who frustrate him. Many youngsters actually believe that their parents are against them and that they mean them no good. This attitude is frequently masked by the phrase "they don't understand me." Their self-destructiveness arises from a deep despair which is unrelated to reality but instead is rooted in pathological processes. Their self-image is commonly distorted to a delusional degree. Accordingly, their impaired judgment is based on such distortions of reality; it is not the result of "immaturity." In fact, they do not learn from experience, because they do not see reality as it is but instead repeatedly subject it to the same distortions which their pathology makes inevitable.

There is a distinct difference between regarding the patient as a sick individual who happens to be an adolescent and viewing him as an adolescent in turmoil who is seeking his "identity," for the process of his illness colors and affects this very effort. In the first instance, we are more likely to be doctors treating the sick (our accustomed role) rather than supportive counselors awaiting the healing effects of time, and tempted thereby to delegate our true function to ancillary professionals. Viewing the early stages of aberrant behavior as mere acting out dulls our clinical acumen. We lose the opportunity to make the proper diagnosis which is so essential to the successful long-term treatment these patients need. Too often, then, parents miss the gravity of what is transpiring and remain aloof from rather than involved in the necessary treatment process.

We find that adolescents respond well in an "adult" program. It would be more accurate to say that they heal well when

treated as sick people among other sick ones who are old enough
to be called adults. Put another way, the young rise to the
occasion when the health in them is uncovered and is encouraged to grow through the measures of isolating and destroying
the disease processes which stunt, fragment, and distort their
efforts at healthy maturation. To our way of thinking, adolescents have adult qualities, just as adults have adolescent ones.
That is to say, patients are a mixture of health and illness.
However, many of the youngsters we see are so very sick and
have been so for so long that little of even the "average adolescent" has had a chance to develop despite the passage of time
which chronologically indicates that they are "adolescents."
When this has been the case, our task is most difficult. It is then
one of creating the earliest kernels of health on which to further
build a maturity consistent with the age of the patient. We are
faced with rearing such patients for the first time through interpersonal experiences they have never had. We assist them to
appreciate what is really transpiring between them and others,
as opposed to what they had imagined to be going on. Our
contention, then, is that a disease process has prevented this
"normal development" and that it is this which requires our
primary attention.

Adolescents in a hospital "act out," as adults do, but in their
own characteristic way. However, they can in most cases relate
to a therapist in typical psychotherapy and profit from it, as well
as family therapy, particularly when supported by drug and
milieu therapy. The patient's hospital life must be structured
carefully and firmly. We find a "closed" facility necessary if the
broad spectrum of adolescent disorders is to be accommodated
for any extended period with a degree of safety. Self-destructive
potential is more to be feared than are destructive and disruptive
capacities. Demands may be made of adolescents, responsibilities placed on them, and restrictions imposed with therapeutic
benefit. Naturally, the timing of these, by whom and how done,
and the setting in which they occur are vitally important to the
success of such tactics.

Factors such as climate, geography, and the availability of
resources will play a part in determining the life of a people. By

the same token, the physical assets and limitations, location, and personnel of an institution will play a part in its social structure and thereby its treatment program. Other factors, of course, will play an important role too. We ourselves had started with a background of experience limited to sick adults. Naturally, we applied our knowledge and thinking derived from it to the adolescent. Housed as we were in one building, necessity permitted us no alternative but to treat the adult and adolescent together. In this vein, then, we all should seek awareness of the correlation between the theories we enunciate and the environment in which we operate and of the correlation between our clinical approach and the uncontrollable factors which influence its espousal. We make this point in the service of objectivity in relating the views and techniques we have developed and justified "on the basis of our clinical experience." Knowledge of this aspect of medicine will help us appreciate the differences we entertain in our concepts of disease and its treatment when there would seem to be no good reason for their existence.

By way of further describing the framework in which our theories of treatment and clinical approach have evolved, we would like to present a short overview of High Point Hospital. Our average census of 40 patients is housed in one building composed of one closed and one open floor, plus two floors for recreational, dining, and office space. We emphasize that it is essential to maintain a *closed* floor. The building is situated on large grounds with all the outdoor recreational facilities usual to such. We think of our total program as a "psychotherapeutic community"—an instrument which in itself has a therapeutic effect. In it our younger patients room, eat, and participate in all ways with the older ones. They are placed in groups appropriate to their symptomatology and behavior, not their age, and given three sessions of psychotherapy per week. Their daily routine is quite similar to that of adults, as is their medication. Our social structure has its own value system, which is brought to bear on patients and staff alike. Its doctors are "active" in their therapy with patients and play a participating role with them in their committee activities and meetings. A major focus of individual treatment sessions is on the patient's difficulties and emotional problems as they relate to his current hospital experience. As these emerge they are related to his earlier and current intrafamilial experiences.

·Having reviewed the history and necessities which prompted and promoted our particular program, and having briefly described our rationale and treatment approach to the adolescent, we would like now to present a statistical report of our experience during the years 1960 through 1964 which compares adolescents and adults with respect to background, clinical and hospital-course factors. This comparison was undertaken to see whether the findings might lend support to our thesis that hospitalized adolescents are in the main mentally sick people who should be treated as such among adults.

By way of describing our sample, then, during the period mentioned, we admitted 92 youngsters aged 14 through 21. We feel justified in including those 19 through 21 as "adolescents" because our patients showed the typical "problems of adolescence," namely, rebellion, regression, problems with identity and with authority, and difficulties in assuming the responsibilities of adulthood. Our data is drawn from their records as well as from those of an equal number of randomly selected adults treated during the same period.

The adolescents had a mean age of 18 years, 5 months and a median age of 19 years, whereas the adults ranged from 23 to 76 with a mean age of 41 years, 10 months and a median age of 39 years, 6 months. There were 42 males and 50 females among the adolescents, and 29 males and 63 females among the adults. Of the adolescents, 72 were at some level of school appropriate to their age, and 85 of the adults were either employed or housewives. Of the adolescents, 88 were single, two married, and two separated, whereas of the adults, 60 were married, 16 single, 9 divorced or separated, and 7 widowed. Of the adolescents, 52 were Jewish, 25 Protestant, 7 Catholic, and 8 of other faiths, whereas of the adults, 49 were Jewish, 22 Protestant, 15 Catholic, and 6 of other faiths; 77 adolescents as compared to 82 adults were "voluntary" admissions.

Graph #1 compares the duration of illness at the time of admission across the two groups; 70 of the 92 adolescents (76 percent) were ill six months or less, whereas 71 of the adults (77

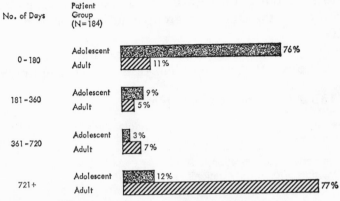

Graph # 1 Duration of Illness Before Admission

percent) were ill two years or more. A "chi" square analysis indicates—as one would expect—a substantially shorter duration of illness in the adolescent population, which is significant at the .001 level of confidence.

Graph #2 compares the type of ambulatory treatment to which each group was exposed prior to hospitalization with us. As would be expected, it shows age-related differences, for younger people generally have both less chance to be sick longer and less chance to have received psychiatric treatment prior to admission. However, it is of interest that the adolescent group,

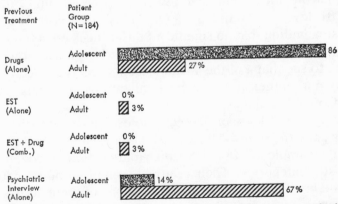

Graph #2 Analysis of Treatment Modalities Prior to Hospitalization (Adolescents receive significantly more drugs. Adults receive significantly more psychotherapy: p<.001)

prior to hospitalization with us, received more drugs and less psychotherapy than the adult group at a significance level of less than .001.

Table 1 compares prior hospital treatment across the two groups. We see that roughly half of each had been previously

Table 1. Prior Hospital Treatment

	Adolescents (N = 44)	Adults (N = 47)
One prior hospitalization	34	12
Multiple prior hospitalizations	10	35

$$\chi^2 = 23.2$$
$$p < .001$$
Adults have significantly more multiple hospitalization

Inpatient Treatment Modalities Administered

EST only	4	4
Drug only	22	19
EST and Drug combined	7	9
No treatment adjuncts	11	15

$$\chi^2 = .73$$
n.s.
No significant differences in treatment agents used.

hospitalized one or more times, again with the age-bound difference that the adolescents had fewer multiple hospitalizations at the .001 level of confidence. One may also note the rather surprising finding that no significant differences emerged in comparing treatment received during prior hospitalizations. It is striking to see that 4 of the 44 adolescents received electroshock therapy during their previous hospitalizations, as compared with four of the 47 adults.

We diagnosed 78 of the 92 adolescents schizophrenic as compared with 60 of the 92 adults. The remaining 46 patients in the total sample of 184 were distributed over a dozen other diagnostic categories. Their relatively small numbers naturally precluded making meaningful comparisons of them across these two groups.

Graph #3, however, compares the remaining large majority of 138 patients (78 adolescents and 60 adults) diagnosed schizo-

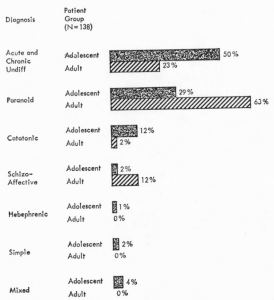

Graph #.3 Comparison of Categories of Schizophrenia (Signifi-cantly more adolescents in Acute-Chronic and Undifferentiated and Catatonic categories. Significantly more adults in Paranoid and Schizo-Affective categories: $p < .001$)

phrenic with respect to "type" of schizophrenia. The following difference emerges at the .001 level: adolescents are more apt to be classified as undifferentiated and catatonic, whereas adults were more apt to fall into the paranoid and schizo-affective categories. Thus, at least in this sample, adults appear to display more of the so-called secondary symptoms of schizophrenia. This difference, however, may also reflect the greater difficulty we have in interpreting adolescent "turmoil" and characteristic "problems with authority" as the paranoid manifestations they often may very well be.

Graph #4 compares the two groups in terms of the frequency with which three treatment adjuvants were used during their treatment at High Point Hospital, namely EST, phenothiazines, and anti-depressants. Note that there were no significant differences in the use of these with either group.

The remaining statistical comparisons presented here will be drawn in some instances between the full adult and adolescent

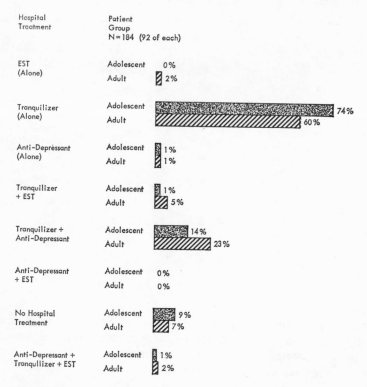

Hospital Treatment	Patient Group N=184 (92 of each)	
EST (Alone)	Adolescent	0%
	Adult	2%
Tranquilizer (Alone)	Adolescent	74%
	Adult	60%
Anti-Depressant (Alone)	Adolescent	1%
	Adult	1%
Tranquilizer + EST	Adolescent	1%
	Adult	5%
Tranquilizer + Anti-Depressant	Adolescent	14%
	Adult	23%
Anti-Depressant + EST	Adolescent	0%
	Adult	0%
No Hospital Treatment	Adolescent	9%
	Adult	7%
Anti-Depressant + Tranquilizer + EST	Adolescent	1%
	Adult	2%

Graph # 4 Type of Treatment Administered During Hospitalization (No significant differences)

samples and in other instances will compare schizophrenic and nonschizophrenic subgroups. Where subsamples are used it is in the interest of comparing treatment response for comparable diagnostic categories. These subsamples were derived by omitting cases in either the adult or adolescent total samples that were not represented in the other group; that is, since there were no chronic brain syndromes or involutional depressions among the adolescents, they were dropped from the subgroup comparisons. Similarly, in the schizophrenic subgroup comparison, only the undifferentiated and paranoid types were retained because the size of the cells for catatonic, schizo-affective, and hebephrenic subtypes were too small to be meaningfully compared.

Graph #5 compares for the two samples the highest "group status" attained while at the hospital. This data is presented as a

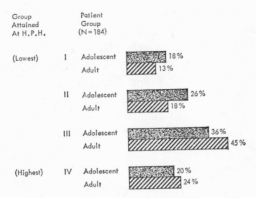

Group Attained At H.P.H.		Patient Group (N = 184)	
(Lowest)	I	Adolescent	18%
		Adult	13%
	II	Adolescent	26%
		Adult	18%
	III	Adolescent	36%
		Adult	45%
(Highest)	IV	Adolescent	20%
		Adult	24%

Graph # 5   Highest Group Attained While at Hospital (No significant differences)

gauge of patient adjustment within the hospital. To understand why we feel that the highest patient group attained is a measure of inhospital adjustment, we must say a few words about how we cluster our patients and determine their status. In short, we place them in succeeding groups, numbered from one to four, each of which exposes them to increasing amounts of interaction, social pressure, privileges, and responsibilities. The medical staff meets each week as a team, together with ancillary professional workers, to evaluate the condition and progress of all patients. At this time it determines the group status of each patient, depending on the reports and opinions of all assembled. Since we are a small institution and are housed in one building, the medical staff gets to know each patient rather well through first-hand contact. Other conferences and means of communication assist in this process. The reports, opinions, and recommendations of the patient's doctor are subject to staff deliberation and consensus is reached. At these conferences we also determine the diagnosis and condition of the patient on discharge.

We are intimately enough in contact with patients to have sufficient confidence in the decisions thus reached in concert. At the same time, from the point of view of statistics, we are mindful that this constitutes a rather crude estimate of clinical movement. However, were there any real differences in inhospital adjustment between the adults and adolescents, one would expect these differences to be reflected in the statistics.

Graph #5, then, compares adolescents and adults with respect to the highest hospital group attained before discharge. As one can see, no significant differences emerge. The highest group achieved by a patient may be thought of as some measure of "within-hospital citizenship" in our institution's scheme of things. Accordingly, adolescents are comparable to adults in their ultimate ability to function at various surveillance and supervision levels, as well as to participate usefully in the communal life of the hospital.

Graph #6 compares the two groups with respect to status on discharge. Note that when the full adult and adolescent samples

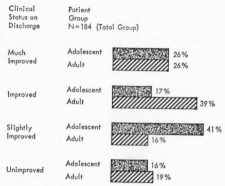

Graph # 6 Clinical Status on Discharge (Significant differences only noted in middle groups: p <.001)

are compared one sees similar or identical numbers of adults and adolescents in the Much Improved and Unimproved categories. A significant difference, however, does emerge in the Improved and Slightly Improved categories, with more of the adults judged as improved. This suggests that among midrange patients, with respect to outcome at time of discharge, adults do somewhat better. However, one is on shaky ground here in interpreting this finding, inasmuch as the adult sample contains 17 fewer schizophrenics but 13 more affective reactions which carry a better prognosis.

However, comparative appraisal of response to hospital treatment would seem to be more meaningful when relatively homogenous entities are compared. Table 2, therefore, com-

Table 2.   Clinical Status at Discharge for Selected Sub-Groups
(Only Non-schizophrenic group approaches significance)

Clinical Status	Non-Schizophrenic (N = 33)		Paranoid Schizophrenic (N = 50)		Acute-Chronic Undifferentiated (N = 55)	
	Adult	Adolescent	Adult	Adolescent	Adult	Adolescent
Much Improved	4	4	10	2	2	14
Improved	7	0	14	3	7	8
Slightly Improved	5	8	5	6	2	12
Unimproved	2	3	8	2	3	7
Total N	18	15	37	13	14	41
	$X^2 = 2.65^*$		$X^2 = 1.78^*$		$X^2 = .14^*$	
	p.11		n.s.		n.s.	

*Categories collapsed for statistical analysis

pares degree of improvement across the two groups for the three major subsamples, namely, the nonschizophrenic, the paranoid schizophrenics, and the undifferentiated schizophrenics. Note that there are no significant differences. Only in the nonschizophrenic subsample does a trend emerge in favor of greater improvement among the adults. But this fails to reach statistical significance.

Table 3 shows a third response factor studied, namely, that of length of stay in the hospital. This factor is difficult to evaluate since it is subject to several extraneous elements such as pressures on adults to return to work or home responsibilities and the family's ability to bear costs. For whatever the statistics are worth, however, full sample comparisons indicate that adolescents stay longer than adults at a .001 level of significance. Note, however, that there is no length-of-stay difference when the two schizophrenic subgroups are compared. Thus the paranoid and

Table 3.   Duration of Hospitalization in Days

No. Days	Total Group (N = 184)		Non-Schizo. (N = 33)		Paranoid (N = 50)		Acute-Chronic Undifferentiated (N = 55)	
	Adult	Adolescent	Adult	Adolescent	Adult	Adolescent	Adult	Adolescent
0–180	67	42	16	8	25	6	11	10
181–360	19	29	1	6	9	6	1	12
361+	6	21	1	1	3	1	2	41
Total N	92	92	18	15	37	13	14	
	$X^2 = 16.15$		$X^2 = 6.01$		$X^2 = 2.23$		$X^2 = 4.46$	
	p. 001		p .05		n.s.		n.s.	

undifferentiated schizophrenics stay just as long, whether they are adolescents or adults. But when the nonpsychotic adolescents and adults are compared, the adolescents are found to stay significantly longer at the .05 level of confidence.

Table 4 shows the actual mean stays for the different subgroups. This raw data is shown only for the sake of comparison with mean stay figures which may be given by other institutions treating adolescents. We realize, however, that mean stay comparisons across institutions are tricky at best insofar as institutional policies and financial and administrative factors may be as apt to determine duration of stay as clinical criteria. In previous graphs we have shown that adolescents in our setting achieve the same group level within the hospital and comparable improvement to their adult counterparts. Table IV indicates, however, that it may take them longer to do so. On the other hand, it may be that their longer hospitalization is less dependent on how well they are doing or the amount of progress they have shown than it is on the lesser demand made on them to return home. Further, there is likely an emotionally based tendency on the part of family to extend itself more for youngsters.

Reviewing the fruits of this statistical survey, we see trends suggestive of the facts that the treatment adjuvants employed in treating adolescents at High Point Hospital do not differ from those used with adults, that adolescents attain comparable levels of good citizenship within the hospital and reach comparable

Table 4. Mean Duration of Hospitalization in Days (Adolescents stay significantly longer as a total group. No significant differences when subjects grouped for diagnostic comparability.)

Group		Total Group (N = 184)	Non-Schizo. (N = 33)	Paranoid Schizo. (N = 50)	Chronic Undiff. (N = 55)
Adolescent	Mean	235.9	173.2	195.2	257.5
	S.D.	221.4	147.8	108.9	247.8
	N=	92	15	13	41
Adult	Mean	142.4	89.6	183.6	147.4
	S.D.	164.8	110.4	208.7	157.7
	N=	92	18	37	14
	t=	3.23	1.86	.25	1.92
	p=	.01	n.s.	n.s.	n.s.

levels of improvement. Except for nonschizophrenic patients, they do this during comparable periods of hospitalization. While a crude statistical survey of this kind cannot be taken as "proof" that adolescents are comparably ill and respond to similar treatment in much the same way as their adult counterparts, these findings nevertheless would appear to lend some measure of support to the validity of such impressions.

Reprint Acknowledgments

Chapter 1 unpublished original.

Chapter 2 reprinted from *The International Journal of Social Psychiatry*, Vol. 14, No. 2, 1968.

Chapter 3 reprinted from *Journal of the National Association of Private Psychiatric Hospitals*, Vol. 2, No. 1 (Spring, 1970).

Chapter 4 reprinted from *Journal of the National Association of Private Psychiatric Hospitals*, Vol. 5, No. 1, 1973.

Chapter 5 reprinted from *Career Directions*, Vol. 2, No. 3, 1971.

Chapter 6 unpublished original.

Chapter 7 reprinted from *Excerpta Medica International Congress Series No. 150*, Proceedings of the Fourth World Congress of Psychiatry, Madrid, September 5–11, 1966.

Chapter 8 reprinted from *American Journal of Psychotherapy*, Vol. 22, No. 3 (July, 1968).

Chapter 9 reprinted from *Hospital and Community Psychiatry*, May, 1969.

Chapter 10 reprinted from *Journal of the National Association of Private Psychiatric Hospitals*, Vol. 2, No. 3, Fall, 1970.

Chapter 11 reprinted from *The Psychiatric Quarterly*, Vol. 45, No. 4, 1971.

Chapter 12 reprinted from *International Journal of Social Psychiatry*, Vol. 21, Nos. 1–2, 1974.

Chapter 13 unpublished original.

Chapter 14 reprinted from *The Psychiatric Quarterly*, January, 1969.

Chapter 15 reprinted from *Behavioral Neuropsychiatry*, Vol. 1, No. 11–12, February–March, 1970.

Chapter 16 reprinted from *Archives of General Psychiatry*, Vol. 20 (March, 1969).

Chapter 17 reprinted from *Archives of General Psychiatry*, Vol. 23 (July, 1970).

Chapter 18 reprinted from *Archives of General Psychiatry*, Vol. 25 (December, 1971).

Chapter 19 reprinted from *Diseases of the Nervous System*, Vol. 30 (December, 1969).

Index

Academy of Psychoanalysis, 153,
157
Acculturation, 8, 10, 153
Ackerman, N. W., 34, 37
Administration, as therapy, 33–
34, 43, 113
Administrator:
psychiatrist as, 118–119
requirements of, in
psychotherapeutic
hospital, 119–120
Adolescents:
abuse of drugs by, 139
concepts of psychopathology
in, 155
as patients at High Point
Hospital, 265–283
problems of, 269
treatment of, 130
turmoil in, 155–156, 270–
271
Alexander, F., 231
American Psychiatric
Association, 48
Arieti, S., 156, 161–164

Billy (case history), 131–133
analysis, 133–134
treatment at High Point
Hospital, 135–137

Blue Cross, regulations
concerning psychiatric
hospital care, 59
Broad-spectrum treatment, 97–
113

Castration anxiety, 99
Caudill, W., 207, 217, 220
Chief authority figure, 73–74
Chronicity, 85–94
Communication, 18–19, 21, 69–
70, 107, 117
at High Point Hospital, 40
therapeutic value of, 108
Community health center, 73
Community psychiatry, 17–18,
54, 99, 147
Countertransference, 37, 93, 111,
123, 126, 128, 163

Disassociated state, 87
Disassociation, 9
Discovery, and development of
mental health, 108

Ego-fragmentation, 270
Electroshock therapy, 55
Essential hypertension, 230
Etzioni, A., 217, 220